Y0-BCF-067

Biomedical Ambiguity

Biomedical Ambiguity

Race, Asthma, and the Contested Meaning of Genetic Research in the Caribbean

Ian Whitmarsh

Cornell University Press
Ithaca and London

Copyright © 2008 by Cornell University
All rights reserved. Except for brief quotations in a review, this book, or
parts thereof, must not be reproduced in any form without permission
in writing from the publisher. For information, address Cornell University Press, Sage House, 512 East State Street, Ithaca, New York 14850.

First published 2008 by Cornell University Press
First printing, Cornell Paperbacks, 2008

Printed in the United States of America

Library of Congress Cataloging-in-Publication Data

Whitmarsh, Ian, 1975–
    Biomedical ambiguity : race, asthma, and the contested meaning of
genetic research in the Caribbean / Ian Whitmarsh.
        p. cm.
    Includes bibliographical references and index.
    ISBN 978-0-8014-4686-3 (cloth : alk. paper) — ISBN 978-0-8014-
7441-5 (pbk. : alk. paper)
    1. Asthma—Social aspects—Barbados. 2. Asthma—Barbados—
Genetic aspects. 3. Health and race—Barbados. 4. Blacks—Health
and hygiene—Barbados. 5. Genetics—Research—Social aspects—
Barbados. 6. Medical anthropology—Barbados. I. Title.
    RA645.A83W45 2008
    362.196'23800972981—dc22
                                        2007051002

Cornell University Press strives to use environmentally responsible suppliers and materials to the fullest extent possible in the publishing of its
books. Such materials include vegetable-based, low-VOC inks and acid-
free papers that are recycled, totally chlorine-free, or partly composed
of nonwood fibers. For further information, visit our website at www.
cornellpress.cornell.edu.

Cloth printing   10 9 8 7 6 5 4 3 2 1
Paperback printing   10 9 8 7 6 5 4 3 2 1

Contents

Acknowledgments   vii

Introduction: Vernaculars in Race and Disease Science   1

1. Contestations of Race   15

2. The Nation as Biomedical Site   33

3. Asthma Variations   56

4. (Re)Categorizing Asthma and the Rational Pharmaceutical   69

5. Biomedical Partnerships: Making Genetics Significant   98

6. Misgivings in Medical Participation   118

7. Participant Mothers   145

8. Home Visit Translations   157

9. Biomedical and Anthropological Excesses   183

Notes   191

References   205

Index   221

Acknowledgments

I am deeply indebted to the families in Barbados who welcomed me into their homes and lives. I thank these mothers and fathers for our interactions. Unfortunately, in order to retain their anonymity I cannot provide names or specify further the families and medical workers who helped me, but I will express particular appreciation to Michael, Suzanne, Harold, Mrs. S., Rosie, Flora, and Enrique. I also thank the genetics researchers and facilitators for their interest in and time with the research, particularly Pissamai, Trevor, and Kathleen.

My colleagues and dissertation advisers at Princeton have made this work what it is. João Biehl had a seemingly endless supply of time and acuity to offer creative, subtle, and productive readings. I thank him for the depth of his commitment to advising and teaching. Chris Garces's friendship and radical interpretations have been invaluable to my project and academic trajectory. Our conversations are reflected throughout this text. Emily Martin was a source of constant strength—in my moments of doubt, her courage and integrity were the clearest signs to me of the value of anthropology. I benefited greatly from Carol Greenhouse's interest in and facility with diverse analytic approaches. Her always close readings of my writings opened new avenues of interpretation of the fieldwork for me. Rena Lederman's subtle interest in subtexts and analytic rigor improved the research greatly. Through his teachings and writings, James Boon has changed the way I think about everything; I'm highly indebted to him. Angela Creager's expansive interest in different disciplinary approaches enriched my understanding of historical trajectories in biology and medicine. Conversations with Michael Oldani on directions in biomedicine have helped me see emerging shifts. I am indebted to Carol Zanca for her help, humor, and warmth. David Jones at MIT and Debra Skinner at the University of North Carolina, Chapel Hill, offered engaging and much needed dialogues about later drafts and interpretations. Other colleagues who have contributed ideas, commentary, and friendship include Sammy Hassan, Chris Roy, Eugene Raikhel, Leo Coleman, and Elizabeth Hough. At Cornell University Press, I especially benefited from thoughtful insights by Peter Wissoker and the extremely helpful anonymous reviewers; I am also grateful to Karen M. Laun, Susan Barnett, and Mary Babcock.

My family has given sustained readings and critical attention to the project, in addition to all the other things family provides. My wife, Jennifer, helped me to attend to moments of ambiguity and ambivalence in my own thinking and in that of my informants. My brother Jason helped me to see underlying ontological and epistemological claims throughout. My sister Megan's approach introduced me to the value of contradictory spaces. My parents, John and Dorothy, have engaged my thoughts with their academic and analytic expertise. To my entire family, those named here and those who have helped in myriad other ways, thank you.

This research was made possible by a grant from the Center for Health and Wellbeing of Princeton University. Preparation of the book was supported by a grant from the Ethical, Legal, and Social Implications Research Program, National Human Genome Research Institute (P20-HG003387) through the Center for Genome Sciences at the University of North Carolina, Chapel Hill, and by a grant from the Andrew W. Mellon Foundation through the Center for the Study of Diversity in Science, Technology, and Medicine at the Massachusetts Institute of Technology. Parts of chapters 2, 4, and 6 are drawn from my article "Biomedical Ambivalence" in *American Ethnologist* 35(1) 2008, published by University of California Press and reprinted courtesy the American Anthropological Association.

Biomedical Ambiguity

Introduction

Vernaculars in Race and Disease Science

The current search for a genetic basis for common illnesses—for example, diabetes, asthma, cancers, depression—is a focus on hereditary susceptibilities. The concept of "biological predispositions" competes with, and draws on, other ways of explaining disease, some more closely related (e.g., characteristics of the blood, "family history," fate) than others (e.g., melancholia, pollution, nutrition, sin). This mix of old and new nosologies is becoming increasingly visible today, as medical geneticists employ racial categories—for example, African American, Hispanic, Caucasian—to make biological links between particular populations and diseases. The terms for these racial categories carry multiple meanings, as do cognate classes including disease categories, medications, and diagnostic techniques, a heterogeneity often masked in the emphasis on the future of medicine. This multivalence is playing an important part in the development of biomedicine today. As scientists, physicians, and patients interact, creating a race-based science of disease, they are constantly translating contrasting approaches to health, ethnicity, and expertise to make the practices of others meaningful. These ambiguities make a race-based science of disease both possible and unstable.

The following pages closely explore a race-based asthma genetics study to see how this science is binding together official and vernacular traditions of identifying ethnic groups and multiple meanings of common illnesses. The study, conducted by a team of researchers from Johns Hopkins

University, was one of six taking place in the eastern Caribbean country of Barbados, a small island with a population of 269,000. Like all such projects, it brought together an otherwise unlikely gathering: the genetics researchers who design and conduct the studies; Barbadian government officials who work to attract international biomedical research; Barbadian medical practitioners and researchers who facilitate data collection; and the families who participate in the study. Through ethnographic fieldwork, I explored what involvement in the research meant to these groups, and the medical and racial categories created through their interaction. This fieldwork revealed foundational contradictions by which those involved both facilitated and potentially undermine the biomedical research program.

This book, then, depicts biomedical research through interviews and ethnographic observations among the multifaceted groups that interact to create such research. The story compels a rethinking of the biomedical stabilization of race and enigmatic illnesses like asthma.

I follow ambiguities by drawing attention to desires, reversals, and contradictory motives—all of which are an integral part of medical science, while often suppressed in representing this science. Giving race and asthma concrete biomedical meaning relies on their historical variability: meanings of race, genes, and asthma are all negotiated in the context of ideas about ethnicity, public health, heredity, and family narratives. The international biomedical research on race and disease is premised on multiple meanings of illness, vernaculars of ethnicity, and national political positions; reciprocally, new medical techniques are produced as this research is integrated into government policies, medical practices, and family identities in surprising ways. The U.S. genomic science occurring in Barbados shows that race-disease connections occurring through biomedical research do not remain on a fixed trajectory; instead they are born with and live a cultural life, creating new regimes of care, state interventions, and unexpected medical diagnostics. This vernacular of medical meanings is integral to the making and use of international genetics of race and disease: its ambiguity allows medical research to have different significance to a postcolonial government, a burdened medical practice, and families.

Variable Asthma

Asthma is an enigmatic condition in American medicine. According to the National Heart, Lung, and Blood Institute (NHLBI), asthma prevalence in the United States increased 75 percent between 1980 and 1994 (NAEPP n.d.). Other research suggests that an increase has occurred worldwide, particularly in urban areas and countries undergoing rapid development. These statistics have elicited various explanations. One of the most common is the "hygiene hypothesis" in which more modern homes and lifestyles result in lower exposure to infections and bacteria at a young age, and a consequent oversensitization to allergens, resulting in asthma. An alternative explanation implicates the increase in pollution associated with modernization. Some epidemiologists argue that increased education, funding, and consequent awareness among both medical practitioners and the public have resulted in a higher rate of diagnosis, not a higher prevalence. A similar explanation notes the expansion of the category of asthma through newer diagnostic techniques such as assessing the response to medications. These competing accounts for the increase reveal a puzzling disease category.

Asthma is a variable object in American and European medical research and practice. As one *Lancet* review of asthma literature states (Tattersfield et al. 2002: 1313), "Asthma has no standard definition." Different diagnostic criteria are employed in both research and medical practice (including response to allergens and medications, self-reporting of symptoms, physician diagnosis, levels of allergen antibodies in the blood and others). In a *Thorax* review of competing measurement practices, the authors (Peat et al. 2001: 406) note, "The difficulty in measuring asthma across populations is that the disease is a complex entity with pathologists, physiologists, clinicians, patients, and epidemiologists all having different perspectives."

The competition between definitions of asthma, methods of measuring it, and ways of categorizing its severity are particularly heightened in the context of the massive funding and research on the condition: the pharmaceutical industry, the World Health Organization (WHO), the NHLBI and Environmental Protection Agency in the United States, and England's National Health Service all offer differing approaches to categorizing and intervening on asthma. Such discordance has historically been foundational to the category's use in British and American medical research: asthma has been neurosis and biology, located in the nerves, the lungs, the blood; caused by dust, pollution, heredity, parental emotions, the unclean farm (overexposure to allergens), the continually cleaned home (underexposure to allergens); treated with stimulants, depressants, steroids, adrenaline, the clean air of the beach, and various tonics. Today, this multiplicity is magnified by the market and medical interest in addressing the growing prevalence. A $24 billion market for respiratory drugs makes asthma investigation a high priority for the pharmaceutical industry, which funds research distinguishing responses to medications, defining the diagnosis of asthma, and measuring its severity. The medical costs of poorly controlled asthma make health care organizations also invest large amounts in asthma management.

Meanings of asthma are shaped through such research and intervention, in an admixture of public and private institutions and techniques. This variation leaves space for competing disciplines and institutions to generate conflicting approaches in categorizing asthma for research and intervention.

The Medical Genetic Future, Presently

The search for genes for asthma is a major endeavor within this field of competition. The NHLBI funds multisited research into the genetics of asthma as a complex disease. Increasingly, the genetics of asthma and of the response to asthma medication (pharmacogenomics) are integrated into single projects: the distinction is blurred as the molecular basis for medication response and disease etiology overlap. As a result, biotechnology and pharmaceutical companies collaborate with academic genetics teams to explore the biological basis for the prevalence and severity of asthma, and the response to major asthma medications.

This collaboration is part of the private and public research into complex diseases and responses to medications occurring as teams search for applications for the vast amount of genomic information generated by genotyping projects.[1] A considerable discussion on the future of genomic-based medicine has accompanied these developments. Media accounts have extensively discussed the potential of "personalized medicine" by which medical regimens will be tailored to an individual's particular genotype[2] and genomic analyses of disease are intended to locate genetic predisposition for common conditions, allowing early pharmaceutical or other clinical interventions.[3]

Genomes in these accounts about the future are configured as sites of technological intervention and scientific research at the forefront of biomedicine. In the gap between this image of the future of medicine and current clinical uses, changes are occurring.[4] My fieldwork began at this juncture, with an interest in the ways genomics made sense of the ambiguities and plurality of "asthma," through the interaction of medical, regulatory, and familial practices. This interest led me to the Washington, D.C., area to look at the regulatory, academic, and private institutions involved in medical genomic research and practice. From July 2002 until July 2003 I interacted with researchers involved in genetics-of-asthma projects; nongovernmental organizations focused on asthma outreach and education; and members of the National Institutes of Health (NIH) and Food and Drug Administration (FDA). My work also included historical research on the medical meanings of asthma at the National Library of Medicine. In conversations with officials and researchers, I was struck by the multiple meanings given to asthma and the enigma of the diverse causes of the condition as well as the level of interest in locating its genetic basis. I also came across the increasing correlation of asthma with biological race.

Vexed Biologies of Race

Pharmacogenomic and genetic medical research is founded on the categorization of populations according to the differential distribution of medically relevant genes. This includes making patient populations genetically representative. In some approaches, the study population is taken to represent disease populations in general: DeCODE's approach in Iceland explores biomedically relevant genes through study of the biological materials and medical records from one country. Other teams pose the prevalence of genetic predisposition as particular to geographically or historically related populations (e.g., Ashkenazi women, African Americans).

In genetics of asthma, populations are classified along ethnic and racial distinctions. This is a robust field, involving funding by the pharmaceutical and biotechnology industries and academic research, and such distinctions were critical to the genetics projects I came across. Several studies have found that African Americans have a slightly higher prevalence of asthma than Caucasians, and a much higher morbidity and mortality rate, and the geneticists I talked with argued that genetic predispositions partially accounted for these disparities. During my fieldwork, I interviewed members of the NHLBI-funded Collaborative Study on Genetics of Asthma (CSGA), which has reported different asthma susceptibility loci among African American, Hispanic, and European American populations. I began to explore the ways the genomic research engaged vernaculars of ethnicity, which, like asthma, had historically contradictory and multiple definitions.

Race is a contested category in biomedicine. Increasingly, racial disparities in the prevalence and severity of diseases are correlated with genetic propensities, and races are differentiated by a genetic basis for response to medication. The biological basis for race has been a troubled object of research over the last century, and today an extensive argument is occurring in medical and scientific journals over the biological basis for race and the utility of race to medicine. Social analyses have critically examined the burgeoning field that relies on long traditions in American concepts of race to make biological claims about health and sickness (see; Lee et al. 2001; Braun 2002; Kaufman and Hall 2003; Kahn 2004; Duster 2005; Shields et al. 2005; Jones and Perlis 2006; Braun et al. 2007; Montoya 2007; Palmié 2007). As a result of this contestation, U.S. regulatory and research practices are attempting to utilize racial classifications that they simultaneously critique.

This conflict is heightened as biomedical research increasingly extends into countries outside the United States and Western Europe.

Chapter 1 follows some of these contradictions in the internationalization of medical research among the FDA, NIH, and academic and pharmaceutical and biotechnology industry projects. I argue that market and moral pressures to address disparities in health are producing an expedient approach to race in which several criteria are each considered independently sufficient for classification. The numerous criteria used to demarcate black race—self-identification on questionnaires, "of African heritage," a set of genes, or attribution by skin color—comprise an integrated set of distinctions. A fundamental slippage is employed such that at times any one can stand for another. Such multiplicity is common to concepts of race, historically and cross-culturally. This variability is constitutive of the efficacy of biomedical racial designations, and the classifications produced by this process are making new populations exchangeable.

Giving Significance to Race-Disease Science

I became interested in the ways this science took on significance: how the ambiguities of race and asthma were constituted by interactions between researchers, medical practitioners, and families. My focus was on a particular research project, in order to follow the mutual translations that occur when families and medical practitioners make use of such bioscience while such bioscience codifies the experiences of families and medical practitioners. During my research in the Washington, D.C., area, I came across an asthma genetics study conducted in Barbados by researchers from the Johns Hopkins Medical School. The Barbados Asthma Genetics Study began in 1993. The study has received the great majority of funding from the NHLBI with some additional funding from a multinational pharmaceutical company. This ongoing project has resulted in the participation of more than 125 families with individuals who have asthma, and the collection of DNA samples and phenotype and questionnaire data on socioeconomic indicators and on the history and severity of asthma. This research has now extended into exploring gene-environment and gene-gene interactions and the genetics of asthma severity and atopy (allergic response). The team has included geneticists, epidemiologists, and clinicians. I became involved with the group through our mutual interest in exploring the current significance of the genetics and pharmacogenetics of asthma and race: I wanted to explore the motives and practices by which international genetics research could occur and had an impact; the team was interested in the ways patients and physicians viewed the genetic research and medical care in

Barbados. From August 2003 to April 2004, I conducted research in Barbados on the Johns Hopkins asthma genetics study, working with the genetics team and Barbadian nurses and physicians who facilitate the project. The genetic research is conducted through home visits in which study facilitators take blood samples, administer an asthma questionnaire, collect dust samples, and conduct spirometry (measuring lung function with an instrument into which patients exhale and inhale). I conducted participant observation during these home visits and at meetings between the genetics team and Barbadian physicians/researchers involved in the studies.

Through this exploration, I examined the ways the Barbadian asthma experience is translated into a genetics of asthma and race, relying on the plurality of "asthma," ethnic identities, and other cultural categories. But my intention was not to conduct a study of a scientific team. Anthropological analyses of science have explored the subjectivities of scientists as they create knowledge and new configurations of scientific, economic, and social trajectories (e.g., see Latour and Woolgar 1979 on the production of scientific concepts; Rabinow 1996 and 1999 on reflexivity in the practice of biotechnology; and Gusterson 1996 on the culture of nuclear scientists). And recent science-studies research has explored the political economy of the science of race and disease (see Kahn 2004; Wailoo and Pemberton 2006). I went to Barbados to examine medical, governmental, and familial practices and interpretations that interact with this science and are integral to its production. I wanted to find what was at stake for the physicians, families, and state officials who formed the infrastructure for the genetics project: the desires and evaluations by which this science is created and has a cultural life, making new medical meanings, national positioning, and patient identities.

Nationalized Biomedicine

The various motives that make Barbados the site of so much biomedical research rely on ethnic designations and state bureaucracy. The country is commonly cited as 92 percent black, and the research is premised on a proposed biological link with other black populations, particularly British and African American ones. Barbados is specifically chosen within the Caribbean because of its extensive national health care system, which provides records and practitioners that facilitate the studies. Medical partnerships are forged between the Barbadian government and U.S. and U.K.-based medical institutions through this nationalized health care system, a process I explore in chapter 2. In interviews with Ministry of Health (MOH) officials, I found that these partnerships comprise part of a public health system that integrates bioscience research and the pharmaceutical industry, making international biomedicine central to disease categorization and health education. This occurs primarily through a national drug formulary, making the multinational pharmaceutical industry critical to health practices. I consequently also conducted interviews with pharmaceutical company representatives and pharmaceutical distributors and producers, and in chapter 2 I explore this amalgamated public and private approach to medical care. Anthropologists have analyzed the role of the multinational pharmaceutical industry in shaping medical perspectives of disease and health (see Petryna et al. 2006; also see Biehl 2004a; Oldani 2004; Lakoff 2005). Pharmaceutical markets play a stronger role in state and medical techniques of health intervention, often marginalizing other public health approaches, in a process of pharmaceuticalization explored by João Biehl (2004a) in the context of AIDS intervention in Brazil. In Barbados, the government frames genomic medical research as a public health practice by linking it with access to the pharmaceutical industry: both are considered forms of participating in global biomedical progress. The genetic research relies on this nationalism.

Increasingly, the discourse on "genetic populations" includes nationhood. The creation of databases around national populations—for example, in Iceland, Estonia, and Sweden—place citizenry at the center of large-scale genomics (Pálsson and Rabinow 2005). As genetic analysis employs national databases of biomedical records and biological samples, governments position their populations for market interventions. Nikolas Rose and Carlos Novas (2005) argue that formations of citizenship are increasingly based on biology: biomedical results are used to give legitimacy and shape to legal, social, and ethnic populations. In Barbados, the government poses the population as biologically black in attracting such international research, reflecting on this vulnerable position in the global economy and its desire to utilize cutting-edge biomedicine. I follow the ways this international biomedical influence is simultaneously a source of pride and distrust among MOH members. Representations of markets and nationhood are employed in exchanges that produce surprising reversals and ironies of pharmaceuticalization. I emphasize the ambiguities at the heart of such global political economic processes that allow them to operate so readily—what in their flexibility is so resilient (on such ambiguities, see Kaplan and Kelly 2000 and Orta 2004).

Collaborative Asthma Diagnoses and Interventions

The market interactions between the pharmaceutical industry and Barbadian government create a robust public health system of research and intervention on the variably defined condition of asthma. Through this mix of industry and government, asthma has emerged in recent years as a biomedical category, drawing on historically contested American and British medical meanings. Before turning to the hybrid of biomedical and traditional diagnostics created around this condition, I pause in chapter 3 to examine the history of this disease, multiply defined with an enigmatic etiology. This chapter traces the variability of asthma in British and American medical research discussed earlier: meanings of heredity, blood, nerves, and treatment have transformed radically over the last two centuries, producing contrasting approaches to asthma. The interventions on asthma in Barbados, including the genetics study, integrate and extend these multiple techniques involved in the diagnosis, categorization, and treatment of an illness.

Barbados is among the countries with the highest levels of asthma in the world, estimated at 18–20 percent of the population. In chapter 4, I explore the significance of these numbers, a documentation produced by the heightened attention from multinational pharmaceutical companies, government intervention, and international biomedical research. I interviewed general practitioners, family doctors, pediatricians, nurses, and pharmacists at polyclinics, at the public hospital, and in private practices who engage an ongoing attempt to standardize a biomedical approach. In Barbados, the integrated variability of asthma (multiple diagnostic criteria used in concert) combines with a pressure to unambiguously diagnose the condition to create an expansive category. The pharmaceutical industry's role in Barbados facilitates this highly inclusive classification along with a resulting emphasis on adherence to medications. Through this adherence discourse, the pharmaceutical has become a rational form of intervention on irrational patients, who take medicine when they want, not when they should. This chapter focuses on the convoluted path of pharmaceuticalization and biomedicalization, as strong criticisms of the overdiagnosis of asthma and overuse of pharmaceutical prescriptions occur alongside their expansion. Various explanations of the high levels of asthma in Barbados based on pollution and diet are used as alternatives to this biomedical understanding. The asthma genetics study takes place within this arena of focused multinational funding, government attention, and practitioner skepticism toward market-based international biomedicine. I argue here that this mix of acceptance and counterdiscourse keeps processes like biomedicalization unstable.

The ambiguities of biomedicine partially run on the interactions between scientists and medical practitioners as expertise is diversely evaluated. In chapter 5, I turn to the fine-grained exchanges between the genetics teams and the Barbadian medical practitioners who provide patients and expertise and collect the materials for the study. The international genetics projects on different diseases in Barbados draw from one another: they share participant populations, Barbadian researchers, and study facilitators. Through these collaborative efforts, genomic databases and patients can be continuing sources of research on new diseases: the existing patient groups, blood samples, and databases generate ongoing potential for studies of new diseases and drug responses. Beneath the simple exchange between American researchers and Barbadian facilitators of records and patient access for technologies and coauthorship, there is a trade in meanings of race, asthma, and expertise. The facilitators work to make the research applicable to Barbados, thereby creating new strategies for dealing with the patient, environment, and illness. Through representations by the genetics team, the medical practitioners come to see Barbadians as biologically linked to African Americans and genetics as the future of biomedicine. The facilitators in turn represent patient populations and environmental factors to the genetics team for new analyses of gene-environment-race-disease. I argue that such exchanges make evaluations of Bajan[5] medical knowledge and U.S.-based genetics expertise integral to the science and medicine produced by the research.

Families Taking Part

These informal exchanges allow the research to produce a black genetic database (for the U.S. team) and a form of state care (for Barbadian officials); they also engender new medical identities. Biological identities are not restricted to use by the state; they are also used and experienced by families. As Adriana Petryna (2002) shows in the context of Chernobyl, these are often hard-won identities, created within regimes of medical access, public health, and open-ended biomedical meanings. In Barbados, the participant families similarly utilize genetic meanings of disease creatively in making sense of the biomedical research and their own conditions. The experiences of participants in genetic research have received some anthropological attention.[6] Rayna Rapp (2003) and Karen Sue Taussig et al. (2003) have explored the ways patient groups become involved in and make genetic research on disorders significant. Margaret Lock (2002) examines the way new market practices become a part of participant evaluation of genomic research. I similarly look to the contrastive and open-ended ways families make meaning of such participation, based on interviews with participants in the asthma genetics study. At the end of home visits, I would explain my research to participant families and ask if they were interested in being interviewed. These conversations often extended to multiple interviews and other interactions, primarily in homes but also at social gatherings.

These families allow researchers and their technologies into their homes to extract blood, measure their breathing, obtain dust samples, and conduct questionnaires. In chapter 6 I explore why. The participants interpret the research based on their experience and evaluations of the national health care system, the expanding diagnostics of asthma, and the pharmaceutical-ization of public health care. Through their involvement, they produce new meanings and interventions on their children's health as they criticize the biomedical link of asthma and pharmaceuticals, and the excess of asthma diagnoses in Barbados. They enact critiques of this system in their decisions to ignore prescriptions, question diagnoses, and look to older kinds of treat-ments. The government and health care focus on adherence to medications is answered with speculations about pharmaceutical side effects. Biomedical models of asthma are questioned with a wealth of posited causes of asthma brought by modernization and international markets (e.g., pesticides, air pollution, imported food). This skepticism toward biomedicalization is wagered within the context of the families' experiences of vagaries of care and fears for their children's health, integrating critique with what is at stake in the daily experiences of illness care. In these practices, families use biomedicine in contradictory and rich ways—hoarding pharmaceuticals rather than consuming them, ridiculing diagnostics that they employ. These evaluations are integral to their participation in the asthma research, which becomes an association with foreign expertise and a rejection of biomedi-calization. The Bajan families forge a medical identity in their participation through a mix of frustration, hope, and doubt about the study results.

In chapter 7, I look to the ways this participation is gendered. Women, as the center of recruitment, are effectively the focal point for the genetics study. I explore what brings mothers particularly to the study—what responsibili-ties, expectations, and identities comprise their experience of being catego-rized as Barbadian mothers of asthmatics. Responsibility for the asthmatic is unambiguously placed with the mother; this message is reinforced in pharma-ceutical marketing pamphlets, in general practitioners' and specialists' state-ments and techniques of care, and among nurses and pharmacists. In the gendered domestic and medical economy, this process results in mothers of asthmatics medicalized as a pharmaceutical facilitator, ambulance substitute, constant monitor, and director of preventive measures. I analyze the ways families engage this role, as a source of pride and frustration. Many women value the study as a form of personalized attention that they consider ab-sent in the public health care system. The contrastive nature of biomedical research in resource-poor countries—valued as foreign—allows the women to use their participation as a response to problematic medical care.

Biomedical Translations

In chapter 8 I turn to the home visit to see the role of these ambiguities and motives within the research. The home visit requires mutual translations, as the researchers produce a science of disease and race out of Bajan experiences and the families make American biomedical expertise and technologies meaningful for their children's conditions. The team must stabilize a plurality of ethnic identities to make the participants "Afro-Caribbean," equivalent to African Americans: Bajan emphases on relational meanings of ethnicity—drawing together nationality, Caribbean heterogeneity, and family histories, with a sense of multiple solidarities—are thereby transformed into biological meanings. Race-disease links are made biological out of this home visit negotiation. In the reciprocal translations by the families, they interpret the foreign and arcane technologies and categories of the genetics researchers. The families maintain this abstract character even as they translate the test results into domestic use. They regard individualized results as valuable personalized attention, despite serving no tangible purpose to their child's condition. I end by exploring what such mutual translations say about the process of creating biomedical (and anthropological) accounts; my argument is that the preclusion of contradiction in such accounts must obfuscate even as it reveals lived experiences and interpretations.

In chapter 9, I suggest some further resonances between what is occurring in Barbados and more broadly in translations of biomedicine across nations, families, and medical practice. The impact of biomedicine occurs through these contexts of patient identity, state categorization of citizenry, and medical practitioner use of genetic meanings. The social interactions that produce these rhetorics—in hospitals, clinics, hotel seminar rooms, patients' homes, public lecture halls, and media outlets—preclude easy distinctions between the production and consumption of biomedicine. The sociality organized around the genomic future results in countries that are unlikely to employ the diagnostic technologies being produced by genetic medicine adjusting their diagnostic techniques, treatment regimens, and local research agendas to align with the perceived biomedical future.

These processes are facilitated with critique, making them foundationally unstable. I explore this open-endedness by following unexpected affinities (for instance, Bajan uses of the word "dust" as an integrated multiplicity, intrinsically vague, like biomedical uses of "race") and contestations (for instance, the simultaneous view of pharmaceutical marketing as a social good and pharmaceuticals as bringing denigrated market-driven care). These ambiguities occur as biomedicine is used obsessively, inconsistently, and culturally, and anthropological attention[6] to such multivalence provides new insights into the extension of international medical markets and discourses.

Contrastive Biomedicine, Contrastive Anthropology

In this book, I avoid adjudicating on the reality of race, genetic predispositions, or asthma: instead, I focus on their use as categories. Following Claude Lévi-Strauss (and Ferdinand de Saussure and Mikhail Bakhtin), medical meanings, like others, are constituted (entirely) by contrast.[7] I here explore the use of race, genes, and disease to constitute medical practices, identities, and scientific knowledges. This use is not reducible to a rational reaction to reality: whether genetic background, disease etiology, the political economy of institutions, or social, economic, or political factors.

As a result, race for the geneticists operates differently than for Bajans, as do "asthma" and "gene." To emphasize this relationality, I explore meanings of "genes," "asthma," "environment," and "Afro-Caribbean" among the genetics team separately from meanings of "wheeze," "genes," "pollution," and racial identity among the Bajan participant families.[8] Genetics is contrasted at some points with immunology, elsewhere with state public health, and elsewhere with pollution research. Asthma is categorized in distinction from, variably, babies wheezing by practitioners and parents, from chronic obstructive pulmonary disorder in medication prescription, from diabetes in models of health education. Race is differently posed as biological, as genetic, as based on self-identification or parental classification, as social, ontological, or strategic in different contexts. I mean here to explore what occurs when these meanings come together: to see how biomedical meanings are translated culturally in ways that play a role in practices organized around the state, illness, science, and care.

My focus is on the multiple motives in utterances and practices I came across.[9] I draw here from anthropological analysis of anomalies—objects that mesh mutually inconsistent cultural categories: for example, Mary Douglas's pangolin (1996), scaly like a fish but land dwelling, allowing it to mediate between spirit, animal, and human worlds; Ralph Bulmer's cassowary (1970), a bird that also represents cross cousins; and Claude Lévi-Strauss's possum (1983) and tortoise (1973), mythic creatures whose anomalous status operates the transformation of nature into culture.[10] These are objects through which people both pronounce cultural distinctions and imagine their alternatives.[11] With the plural uses of these anomalies, cultural values are simultaneously experienced, made real, and questioned. Throughout, this work looks to the uses of diagnostics, of pharmaceuticals, of disease, of food, to find such anomalous objects, to see the ways biomedical categories are simultaneously questioned and effected. I explore categories and things (including scientific, technological, capitalist, and medical ones) as made and used in mutually inconsistent ways.

Part of this plurality is ambivalence: I became interested in the ways that biomedical practices such as genomic research, pharmaceuticalization of health, and the link between race and disease were simultaneously valued and critiqued within the logics I encountered. Geneticists, Bajan families, medical practitioners, and state officials all expressed conflicting evaluations and conceptualizations of the practices in which they were involved: for example, internationalism could be a source of pride and bitterness, biomedical categories could be laughed at and utilized, and medical identities could be contradictory. These moments of ambiguity and reflexivity seemed to be critical to the creation and implementation of biomedical meanings of "race" and "asthma." These contradictions are not simple reflections of political economies (whether of institutions, knowledge, or affect). I mean here to search out what James Boon (1998: 65) calls "resonant details," moments of irony, of anomaly, of surprising connections and reversals by which meaning is made. My argument is that the ambivalent interpretation of processes like pharmaceuticalization and biomedicalization found among those engaging in them—officials, physicians, patients—is central to both their entrenchment and instability.

This is an exploration of the biomedical vernacular: the ways genetics, asthma, race, nation, and environment are used culturally, and the mutual extremes and excesses that make such meanings contradictory. The relationship of such vernaculars (including those of officials) to official discourses (including anthropology's) is a vexing problem. I mean here to give an account of the ways discourses determine political economies, mute alternatives, the way identities are made of such categories, while being attentive to the way people are not fixed within these logics, that categories include the possibility of their negation, that cultures, families, individuals, and communities reflect on their categories in excesses that cannot be contained in any analytic approach. This book is an attempt to oscillate between these contradictory emphases rather than choose one or blend them into a consistent whole.

Chapter 1

Contestations of Race

Race is a thorny topic in American biomedicine today. As Morris Foster and Richard Sharp (2002) have argued, the Human Genome Project created interest in new applications of the relationship between genetic predispositions and race. A growing body of research attempts to link racial disparities in the prevalence and severity of diseases—for example, cancer, heart disease, asthma—with genetic propensities. The genetic basis for response to medication—including genes involved in drug-metabolizing enzymes and chemotherapeutics—has been similarly differentiated by racial categories. The Food and Drug Administration (FDA) has recently approved a heart medication, BiDil, that is the first pharmaceutical produced for and marketable to a particular racial group (see Kahn 2004 for a subtle discussion of the development of BiDil). The approval of BiDil, as with other projects based on purported biological differences between races conducted by the pharmaceutical and biotechnology industries and NIH-sponsored academic teams, has resulted in contentions over whether biological races exist, and if so, whether such categorization is medically relevant.[1] The contested field of race in bioscience is exacerbated by the increasing trend toward international biomedical research. As the FDA, NIH, and the pharmaceutical industry attempt to incorporate the results of this research, new links are being made between racial groups in the United States and populations in

Japan, the Middle East, Africa, and Latin America. The multiplicity of race is constitutive of this extension of biomedical work.

Race as Biological

Critics have argued that biological meanings of race should not be used in medical research. Many note the often-cited conclusion that greater genetic variation exists within groups than between them (Jenny Reardon (2005: 35) traces this datum, now found by many studies, to biologist Richard Lewontin). Craig Venter, the founder of the company that led the private sector's role in sequencing the human genome, uses this conclusion to argue against the use of race in clinical trials, in favor of an individualized approach (Haga and Venter 2003). Shields et al. (2005) argue that more precise ways of defining populations to study disease are available that obviate the need for self-identified race as a proxy for biological connections in biomedicine. Others point to the problems resulting from correlations of race with disease. Lee et al. (2001) and others (Duster 2003; Foster 2003) argue that the one-to-one association of sickle cell anemia with black race resulted in discriminatory mandatory testing policies and underdiagnosis of white patients with the disease.[2] The potential for discrimination in medical care has also been raised with the current heart medication research: two health care industry consultants found evidence that physicians incorrectly interpreted the research to mean that black patients should not be prescribed the heart medication angiotensin-converting enzyme (ACE) inhibitors (Masoudi and Havranek 2001). Biomedical researchers have responded to these critiques of the use of biological race in medicine by arguing for the necessity of accounting for all of the causes, genetic or otherwise, in the disparities in disease prevalence and severity between different races.

Such debates, in the *Journal of the American Medical Association, Nature,* the *New England Journal of Medicine, Lancet,* and other medical and scientific journals, often draw on studies by population geneticists who categorize races on the basis of genetic frequencies. In this research on genetic diversity, groups are selected as racially distinct, and differences in genetic frequency are studied. Population geneticists, as Reardon (2005) has shown, disagree on how best to categorize race. Determining the race of the population being studied is one such source of dispute (Rosenberg et al. 2002: 298): for example, self-reporting is contrasted with inferring ancestry through genotyping. Additionally, these projects usually involve populations from different countries, and which categories are applicable, particularly in the case of Caucasian, is disputed. Population geneticists also disagree over the genes to be used, with some advocating particularly informative genetic markers and others arguing for randomly selected genes. Such categories rely on concepts of purity in an imagined past, as populations are measured according to an admixture of race-specific genes—for example, the amount of European genes in African Americans (Esteban et al. 1998; Graves 2001: 201–3). These posited distinct histories are also considered significant for study design, as more "recently admixed populations" are understood to provide different kinds of information than do groups considered more genetically distinct (Esteban et al. 1998). One of the generally accepted conclusions of this research is that Africa has the largest amount of genetic variability, due to the history of the human population.

Population genetic research on human diversity is variably incorporated into discussions about the use of race in biomedicine. There is a discourse arguing for the integration of geographic ancestry research into biomedical diagnostics of race and disease (anthropologist Duana Fullwiley is tracking the inclusion of a particular technology to conduct such research). These geneticists debate whether races that are distinguishable by particular genetic markers would be distinguishable by biomedically relevant genes (on this debate, see, e.g., Jorde et al. 2001; Wilson et al. 2001; Romualdi et al. 2002). But most agree on employing evolutionary history and population genetics in current biomedical research. Mark Shriver is an anthropologist whose research purports to correlate skin color and self-identification with genetic admixture of European, African, and other sources of ancestry; he uses his research to try to locate biological bases for differences in disease prevalence between races (Gower et al. 2003). Genaissance is a biotechnology company working on pharmacogenomics that particularly advocates such analysis. In an article in *Science* comparing genetic variability between populations labeled Hispanic Latino, African American, and Caucasian, Genaissance researchers argued for the use of self-reporting of race for genomic medicine, concluding, "Our observations demonstrate the necessity of understanding patterns of human genomic evolution if genomic variability is to be used as a tool in human health research" (Stephens et al. 2001: 492).

However, such use of genetic diversity research in biomedical disputes over race is rare. In my experience, researchers working on the genetics of diseases and the pharmacogenetics of drug responses employ racial distinctions largely independent of studies on genetic ancestry and diversity. Some of the results of such research are deployed: the datum that Africans have the greatest genetic variability is frequently used in support of genetic research on people of African descent as being particularly informative. But biomedical research and genetic diversity projects have differing perspectives on the purpose and method of defining races. One biomedical researcher explained to me the difficulties that Genaissance was having in attracting interest among pharmaceutical companies with its population history approach. Genetic diversity research involves categorizing human populations by geographic areas and specific genetic loci chosen for their correlation with these areas; such focused designations of race, geographic origin, and genetic markers are of little use to most medical researchers and of less use to practitioners. In medical research, the genetic history of a population analyzed by human diversity geneticists is at times invoked, but this operates as a kind of atemporal history used to speculate about results rather than as an organic variable that produces new research questions. Instead, biomedical research primarily examines differentiation in medically relevant genes between races identified through more traditional means. These researchers most often use a utilitarian definition, based on the racial meanings employed in the census, geographic site of research, physical appearance, or the participants' own identification on a questionnaire. This production of race-disease links draws on historical, medical, and scientific meanings of race. The categories deployed—such as Asian, African American, Caucasian—emerge out of this historical complexity, informing the current biomedical use of the genetics of populations. The anthropological interest, then, is to find not the meaning of race in biosciences, but rather the techniques by which race can have so many meanings in bioscience. Race gains its facility as a relational discourse in exchange with other meanings and categories. Biological meanings of race draw from social, cultural, and economic ones.

The Medicine of Race, Blood, Disease

As Waltraud Ernst (1999b) points out, the ambiguities and contradictions in ideas of race have historically been a source of the concept's strength within science. Historian Nancy Stepan (1982) shows that the science of race in the nineteenth century created hierarchies of, variably, Africans, Mediterraneans, Jews, Caucasians, Asiatic, gypsies, and other groups. Racial theories were also used to constitute political legitimacy of nation-states as Western Europe was divided into the racial types of Celts and Anglo-Saxons, Gauls and Franks, Germans and Slavs (Augstein 1999).[3] This relational character of racial classification—its ability to integrate divergent, sometimes contradictory contents—has been foundational to its extensive scientific and medical use.[4] Race in this sense has a valued polysemy. This variability was belied by highly precise and technological measurements in the nineteenth-century science of race; for example, skull measurements were used to give exact numbers on intellect, moral worth, capacity for civilization, level of spirituality, cultural complexity, technological sophistication, and so on. The result was a science that examines visibly physical characteristics as constituting historical trajectories of biologically distinguishable populations. Race was in the blood in this nineteenth-century science, carrying taboos of mixing and association with disease in perspectives on immigrants, populations in the colonies, and those considered black in the United States (see Banton 2000; Foucault 2003; and Khan 2004).[5] The particular content of each classification—which groups were included—has been less stable than this emphasis on precise measurements of a characteristic carrying multiple associations.

In the twentieth-century United States, the scientific link between blood, race, and disease became genetic. In the 1920s and 1930s, the genetics of race was mutually constituted with the genetics of disease. Daniel Kevles (1995) shows that racial distinctions were considered significant to human genetics from the inception of the field. Racially mixed populations were valued as genetically variable, taking the (conceptual) place of hybrids made in controlled experiments (193). This mixing relied on the idea of pure groups, whether as abstract ideal populations or as in existence somewhere (i.e., the races prior to or unaffected by hybridization). The scientific interest in the genetics of racial subgroups helped generate the emerging human genetics. For example, in Kevles's account, the genetics of blood groups (worked out in 1911) became an object of extensive research only in the 1930s through the differentiation of races by blood group frequency (195). Race was positioned with twin and family studies as sources of particular genetic knowledge:

> In 1931 [...Lancelot] Hogben called for the establishment of what amounted to a multi-part human genetic research program: twin studies to sort out the relative roles of heredity and environment; measurements of variability within hybrid populations to test for "race"-specific characters; pedigree investigations, especially from medical records, for determining the genetic basis of disease; and surveys of consanguinity, to decide whether certain diseases or physical traits might be the product of homozygous recessives. (198)

This type of a diagnostics of race reframed former meanings, geneticizing the blood-race links, pure races, and the associations of disease and race.[6]

In the United States, the clearest association of blood, race, disease, and genetics in the early twentieth century was sickle cell anemia. Keith Wailoo

(1997: 134–61) shows the ways that Mendelian genetics was used in the 1920s to shape the meaning of sickle cell anemia as a "potential disease" within "negro blood." Such links made between diseases, races, blood, and heredity were implicated in brutal practices toward particular populations, as Wailoo, Kevles, and others have documented, including in immigrant sterilization and other eugenics programs (Kevles 1995), medical discrimination (Wailoo 1997), and in the Tuskegee study on syphilis (see Jones 1981).

In the 1940s, the association of race research with Nazism resulted in changes in science in the United States. In her historical analysis of race in twentieth-century science, Reardon (2005) shows that new moral and political stances were taken in opposition to the association of racial distinctions with moral and mental hierarchies. Population geneticists distinguished their work from political implications that were no longer tenable in the climate of the United States. Reardon points out that these shifts did not include a widespread rejection of a biological basis for racial distinctions, but instead geneticists and anthropologists attempted to delineate more precisely the biological meaning of race. The genetic links of blood, race, and disease became an explicit object of evaluation in this process. Debates about the biological basis for race in the middle of the century emphasized the moral meaning of these methodological quandaries of racial categorization.

Moral Analytics

In 1962, Frank Livingstone (1962: 279) made his much-cited comment, "There are no races, there are only clines." In the discussion that followed this statement over the next two years in the pages of *Current Anthropology*, the moral, ontological, and strategic meanings of race were explicitly placed in opposition.

This discussion continued anthropological arguments over the physiological basis for race going back to the late nineteenth century.[7] Franz Boas radically destabilized contemporary concepts of race as a linguistic, cultural, and even physiological entity with his research on language; cultural change; and changes in body shape among immigrants toward U.S. norms. He wrote:

> Added to this is the failure to see that the many different constitutional types composing a race cannot be considered as absolutely permanent, but that the physiological and psychological reactions of the body are in a constant state of flux according to the outer and inner circumstances in which the organism finds itself. (Boas 1983: 255)

Faye Harrison (1995: 54) notes that Boas was not alone in conducting such research critiquing the science of race that linked mental and physiological characteristics; his work was complemented by that of other anthropological researchers. Boas's students subsequently took up such positions. Ashley Montagu's anthropologically influential work, *Man's Most Dangerous Myth* (1997), similarly extended critiques of the biological, intellectual, linguistic, and cultural characteristics grouped under the term "race."[8]

Theodosius Dobzhansky (1962) responded to Livingstone's statement by arguing that the quandary was a problem of nomenclature. For Dobzhansky, racial classifications were analytic designations, distinct from the ontological existence of races (which was indisputable): "There is nothing arbitrary about whether race differences do or do not exist, but whether races should or should not be named, and if they should, how many should be recognized, is a matter of convenience and hence of judgment" (280). Dobzhansky's framing restricted arguments against the use of race to whether particular terminologies should (morally, socially, occasionally scientifically) be employed.[9] When Livingstone responded to this formulation (1963), he emphasized the historical and cultural meanings that, he maintained, infused this proposed ontology. He drew attention to the socially significant types of racial classifications that were consistently made: "It is curious that we haven't yet discovered the valid races of Europe although perhaps more is known about these populations than any others. But the implication remains that if we keep collecting data, we will someday discover how many races there are in Europe. I don't believe it" (200). This positioning of race as an ontological, epistemological, or nomenclatural problem was taken up in subsequent anthropological encounters. Two years later, a series of responses between geneticists and anthropologists in *Current Anthropology* extended the discussion between Livingstone and Dobzhansky. C. L. Brace (1964) offered support of Livingstone's perspective. Carleton Coon (1964: 314), whose work on race brought considerable criticism from Montagu (see Montagu 1963a), argued that boundaries between races did not need to be arbitrary if "one considers the existence of racially intermediate zones as separate categories." Earl Count (1964: 315) argued that "'trait' varies in meaning under atomistic, typological, populational, processural, configurational thinking." At stake here was the question of the significance of race as a methodological tool, a physical reality, and a scientific designation.

This moral and epistemological contestation over the scientific uses of race is today integral to debates in biomedicine. One could trace the issue of racial physiological classification schemas as epistemological or ontological at least to Georges-Louis Leclerc de Buffon and Carolus von Linnaeus.

What is particular to the discussion above is the explicit interweaving of scientific, political, and medical meanings, by which moral claims could be made. Dobzhansky (1962: 280) ended his response to Livingstone by invoking the morality of the debate: "To say that mankind has no races plays into hands of race bigots, and this is least of all desirable when the 'scientific' racism attempts to rear its ugly head." In Livingstone's response, he also positioned the dispute morally, although differently: he argued that the high frequency of diseases such as sickle cell anemia among Turks, Africans, Indians, and others had a different explanation (natural selection) than other traits that are shared through historical links, making racial classification inextricable from its former associations (1963: 199–200). Today, biomedical approaches to race and health similarly emphasize the moral meanings of race as an epistemology and ontology. This ethical significance takes the form of medical need, social redress, and political implementation.

Urgent Science

The science of race and disease has produced a wealth of literature correlating race with disparities in disease prevalence, diagnosis, treatment, and mortality and morbidity rates (Graves 2001; Committee on Understanding and Eliminating Racial and Ethnic Disparities in Health Care 2002; Good et al. 2002). For instance, African Americans have higher mortality rates for tuberculosis, diabetes, pneumonia, ulcers, and heart disease (Graves 2001). Researchers have shown disparities in health insurance, health care delivery and availability, and exposure to hazardous waste and environmental toxins (Graves 2001; Smedley et al. 2003). African Americans and Hispanic populations have been found to have higher rates of asthma in the United States, with considerably higher morbidity and mortality rates (NCHS n.d.; Nsieh-Jefferson 2003).

These disparities give a moral significance to genetic research on race and disease. The geneticists I talked with frame their projects in terms of intervention on such disparities, through the localization of particular genetic predisposition to disease or to discern medications that are particularly effective among minorities (see Shields et al. 2005 for a multidisciplinary discussion of this framing). Including racial or ethnic groups in genetics research is often thought to be important both by geneticists and by individuals considered representative of ethnic communities (e.g., see Reardon's 2005 discussion of the Genomic Research in African American Pedigrees project (G-RAP) designed by Howard University geneticists and biostatisticians, intended to create a linkage map of African American genomes).[10]

Medical markets are also critical to this gene-race-disease research. Such research combines the moral agenda of redressing disparities with the economic value of having access to genomic databases, biological samples, patients, and medication target populations. This market and moral interest gives gene-race-disease research an urgency. Regulatory, commercial, and research institutions in this context create a fractured approach to race.

In the United States, this contestation occurs primarily through government and private institutions interested in categorizing populations for medical intervention, such as the NIH, FDA, and pharmaceutical industry. In recent years, each of these institutions has contended with conflicting approaches to racial categories. These spaces of public ambiguity have opened through increasing emphasis by the social sciences on race as socially constructed; increasing pressures to address minority disparities in health; and the move to conduct biomedical research in countries outside the United States and Western Europe, resulting in the quandary of how to make populations of resource-poor countries representative of U.S. and U.K. populations.

NIH on Race

Ambiguities in the biomedical uses of race are highly visible in NIH practices. Since 1993, with the Revitalization Act, the NIH has had a policy advocating the inclusion of "women and members of racial and ethnic groups" in clinical research (see Reardon 2005). Sandra Lee, Joanna Mountain, and Barbara Koenig (2001: 42)[11] note that the NIH uses the racial classification scheme of the Office of Management and Budget (OMB), also used by the U.S. Census Bureau (see also Shields et al. 2005). However, the OMB (as these authors point out) considers race and ethnicity categories sociocultural constructs, in accordance with the suggestions of the American Anthropological Association. The result of these policies has been a diversity of views of race and ethnicity in NIH-funded research. Owing to the policy of considering race a social cultural construct, researchers applying for NIH funding almost ubiquitously use the term "ethnicity" instead of "race." Ethnicity in this sense usually involves self-identification on a questionnaire as one of the U.S. census populations, and the uses of this identification in research vary from biological to social meanings in NIH-funded projects (Lee et al. 2001; on the radical variation in methods of determining race in biomedical research, see Shanawani et al. 2006). Contradictory meanings of race are thereby incorporated into policy and practice. The National Human Genome Research Institute's Haplotype Map (Hapmap) project, for example, is a collaborative effort that collected genotype information from three populations taken to be representative of different ethnicities—ninety individuals in Utah, ninety in East Asia, and ninety in West Africa—in an attempt to identify large blocs of genetic markers that can be used to facilitate biomedical research. Medical genetic researchers use this database to analyze their data—for example, excluding particular individuals from their analysis because they are genetically shown to be "of non-European ancestry" based on genotypic comparison with the Hapmap data (see, e.g., Wellcome Trust Case Control Consortium 2007). As a result of these contingencies of practice, ethnicity often becomes a biological entity with medical relevance in medical literature. These uses of "race" and "ethnicity" operate distinctly from the evolutionary history of genetic diversity research. Instead, self-identification by questionnaire is taken to more or less represent biological differences between populations, and the disputed question is whether a particular disease is influenced by such differentiation.

FDA on Race

This contradictory set of approaches to race is also found in medical regulation. In 1998, the FDA began requiring pharmaceutical companies to submit analyses of safety and effectiveness in "racial subgroups" for all new drug applications (Temple 2002). In 2003, the FDA issued a document entitled "Guidance for Industry: Collection of Race and Ethnicity Data in Clinical Trials." These principles are not legal responsibilities, but they are highly influential in the collaborative process between the pharmaceutical industry and FDA of getting drugs to market. The document is specifically designed to account for the changes occurring as a result of the trend of clinical trials being conducted in other (generally poor) countries through contract research organizations (see Petryna 2005 for an exploration of this phenomenon). Given the FDA's role of regulating medicines for U.S. consumption, this shift has caused concerns at the FDA over whether these populations are ethnically representative of U.S. populations.

In the Guidance document, the FDA reiterates the OMB's stance on race:

> The OMB stated that its race and ethnicity categories were non-anthropologic (in other words, not scientifically based) designations but, instead, were categories that described the sociocultural constructs of our society. (Food and Drug Administration 2003)

The document goes on to list various physiological and biological racial distinctions that are considered medically relevant:

> For example, in the US, Whites are more likely than persons of Asian and African heritage to have abnormally low levels of an important enzyme (CYP2D6) that metabolizes drugs belonging to a variety of therapeutic areas, such as antidepressants, antipsychotics, and beta blockers....Additionally, after using some drugs in the psychotherapeutic class, slower enzyme metabolism (CYP2C19) has been observed in persons in the US of Asian descent as compared to Whites and Blacks.

In contemporary federal approaches to biomedicine, race holds these contradictory roles as socially constructed, not scientifically based, but differentiable by genetic research into drug responses.

The Guidance recommends that companies conducting clinical trials use the OMB list for collecting race information: American Indian or Alaska Native; Asian; black or African American; Native Hawaiian or Other Pacific Islander; and white. To accommodate the trend toward clinical trials in other countries, the FDA suggests that "more detailed categorizations of race and ethnicity" can be used—for example, European, Middle Eastern, or North African for white; or Indian or Japanese for Asian. Race is thereby positioned variably as geographic, biological, and social. The Guidance notes that "if sponsors choose to use more detailed characterizations of race and ethnicity, it is important for analytical purposes that the data trace back to the recommended categories described below." These categories are identical to the previous list (above) except in place of "Black or African American," is written "Black, of African Heritage." Here, the FDA contends with the biomedical vagaries of race/ethnicity. Race in this regulatory framework becomes variably cultural, biological, and medical, often in mutually exclusive forms.

This multiplicity has resulted in institutional friction. In March of 2003, the pharmaceutical industry trade organization PhRMA issued a response to the FDA Guidance. Their response focuses particularly on the discrepancies of race as cultural and as biological:

> It is stated that the OMB race and ethnicity categories were not scientifically based designations but instead, were categories describing the sociocultural construct of society in the USA. In the next paragraph, OMB categories are proposed as appropriate for evaluation of the influence of intrinsic factors, such as genetic factors. (PhRMA 2003)

The response identifies several categorical problems with the Guidance. PhRMA argues that some populations remain ambiguously categorized (e.g., Laplanders, Maori) and some racial groups are too broad (e.g., Asian). The response refers to the category white as "US-centric," not mapping well onto the more commonly internationally used "Caucasian," which includes the people of northern India. In contrast to this taxonomy, PhRMA repeatedly posits the need for scientifically based race and ethnicity categories.

These ambiguities and contestations reveal the ways race and ethnicity are being posited in biomedical practice through particular projects. In contrast to genetic variability research, the categories of race and ethnicity in biomedicine are being shaped by the sites chosen by contract research organizations for clinical trial markets; FDA understandings of pharmacogenetic research; and NIH-sponsored explorations of genetics of disease. As such research extends into various countries, new links are made between disease populations.

This contingency in practice has resulted in the varied use of racial categories and disease. Biomedical research has attempted to differentiate several genetic predispositions by racial prevalence. For example, genetic precursors to type II diabetes and to osteoporosis have been associated with racial categories, as have various genes involved in drug metabolism. Pharmacogenetic studies have found that Asians and Africans have an allelic variant in the gene encoding glucose-6-phosphate dehydrogenase that affects reaction to the antimalarial primaquine, in addition to other drugs (Lowitt and Shear 2001; Omenn and Motulsky 2003); approximately 50 percent of Caucasians compared with 80 percent of Egyptian peoples are reported to have a variant of the N-acetyltransferase-2 (NAT-2) gene that can cause an accumulation of toxic levels of isoniazid, a drug used to treat tuberculosis (Lowitt and Shear 2001); several polymorphisms of genes coding for the cytochrome p450 (CYP450) proteins are differentially correlated with being Asian, African, or Caucasian (Rusnak et al. 2001); and the FDA has approved a glaucoma drug that is marketable as being more effective in black patients (Lee et al. 2001). These statistics and research practices are producing new groupings of international populations.

Hyperdiagnostics of Race

The moral and market dimensions of race-disease links create a pressure to stabilize concepts like race for medical intervention. This creates a kind of expedient pragmatics to the biology of race that considers skin color, self-identification, parental ethnicity, and geographic ancestry (inferred or stated) each as diagnostic of race. The precise differences between these criteria for identifying race are not viewed as important to discern, in the need to treat people. The pressure exerted by markets and the sense of moral urgency is not to become consistent but to become efficacious, and in the case of race science, multiple forms of race identification used expediently produce results.

Biomedicine, then, like other approaches, treats race as *simultaneously* biological, medical, geographic, and socially constructed. But unlike other approaches, this allowance of a vague grouping along inexact lines collapses once results are found—for example, at the point where one needs to consider Japanese as representative or not representative of U.S. populations in order to sell pharmaceuticals or to develop medical routines. When this expedient approach to race combines with the diagnostic technologies of biomedicine, the result is a hyperspecific measurement of the highly variable object of race: e.g., 50 percent of Caucasians with the NAT-2 gene, and percentage of genetic Hispanic admixture. This radical precision of measurement applied to a constantly shifting category is a kind of hyperdiagnostics of race.

This strange quality of race in bioscience today is illuminated by Michel Foucault's work. In *The Order of Things* (1994a), Foucault argues that the table became the organizing tool of knowledge in the seventeenth and eighteenth centuries. Linnaeus's classificatory system as a table was a set of identities and differences by which all objects could be placed into a grid. Beings represented in this table lacked a history, or had a history without movement.[12] The physical characteristics that were used to calculate difference and similarity were independent of their historical trajectories or significance. Instead of locating functional or historical links or divergences, according to Foucault, the table offered the name: the name signified the identities and differences with other objects in the table—that is, it placed the being in the grid.

The critical insight that Foucault offers is that this form of knowledge had a contradictory function: it was both a self-consciously constructed tool—Linnaeus created the "Method" reflexively to organize beings—and a signifier of ontology, since all beings only existed within the table (i.e., through representation). Therefore, representation, which was analyzed for efficacy, parity, and direction by discourse, was also a frame that contained all things within it. As Foucault puts it:

[To make use of signs] is an attempt to discover the arbitrary language that will authorize the deployment of nature within its space, the final terms of its analysis and the laws of its composition. It is no longer the task of knowledge to dig out the ancient Word from the unknown places where it may be hidden; its job now is to fabricate a language, and to fabricate it well—so that, as an instrument of analysis and combination, it will really be the language of calculation. (1994a: 62–63)

In this practice, representation takes on the qualities (simultaneously) of reflexive falsehoods (or approximations/models) and direct truths.

The uses of race in bioscience today carry this same uneasy quality: racial categories are posed as ontological because they are genetic, strategic because they are a step toward obviating their use, and socially constructed. And, like Foucault's table, they are taken to depict reality: the table can be used for diagnosis, medical intervention, and genealogy.

Stabilizing Contingency in Heart Research

BiDil illustrates this approach. BiDil is a combination of two previously available heart medications that was originally developed by a company called Medco Research. After failing to get approval by the FDA, the drug was subsequently picked up by the company NitroMed working with the Association of Black Cardiologists (Kahn 2004). In 2005, NitroMed got approval from the FDA to market the product specifically for the treatment of black patients. Jonathan Kahn (2004) has tracked the interplay of legal and commercial practices by which this pharmaceutical "became ethnic." His detailed analysis examines the way racial categorization is often added retrospectively in medical science. The primary incentives for this development of BiDil were the widespread biomedical conclusions that 1) black patients have higher levels of heart failure than other populations and 2) black patients respond poorly to two major classes of heart medications—beta blockers and ACE inhibitors—in comparison with white patients (Exner et al. 2001; see Kahn 2004 for a critique and qualification of both of these claims). The literature that reaches these conclusions illustrates the significance of race for biomedical researchers. As medical outcomes are differentiated by race, the causes of the outcomes are open to interpretation: genetic, physiological, economic, and access to medical care are all noted as potential causes of disease disparities. An interaction of these factors is usually posited. Hence, the biological becomes one of several aspects of race. With this formulation it becomes unnecessary to precisely define race or the contribution of genes to health: biological race can be substituted for social race because outcomes are the only area considered relevant.

The other primary function of race in the research on heart conditions is as a proxy. Researchers speak repeatedly of the use of race for biomedical research as an intermediate step to finding particular genetic populations— that is, toward eradicating the necessity of using race in biomedicine. Race is referred to as a "place holder" or a "surrogate marker." It becomes a strategic practice, rather than an ontological entity, reminiscent of the arguments in *Current Anthropology* discussed earlier. The significant point is that the concept of race as a tool becomes a necessary step toward future research: the direction of biomedicine is invoked as requiring such a proxy.[13] In this sense, attention in biomedicine is directed toward the future, which will obviate the problematics of current techniques but only through their contemporary utilization.

The anthropological question amid the discussion of potential and the future of genetic medicine then is, what is occurring in this contemporary utilization? To see the effects, and uses, and critiques of racial categories we need to listen to the ways researchers, practitioners, and families are taking up particular findings.

Asthma, Race, and Genetics

The genetics of asthma and asthma medication response is a large and varied field of research. Geneticists view asthma as a multifactorial disease, caused by several genes in interaction with the environment, resulting in studies focusing on various genetic loci and environmental factors. Race is a critical component of much of this research. Several epidemiological studies have made the case that African Americans have a slightly higher prevalence of asthma than Caucasians, and a much higher morbidity and mortality rate (Lang and Polansky 1994; Eisner et al. 2000; Miller 2000; Rona 2000). According to the Centers for Disease Control and Prevention (CDC), African Americans are three times more likely to be hospitalized or die from asthma (NCHS n.d.). Some studies have found that African Americans and Hispanics are more likely to have asthma after controlling for income and other socioeconomic indicators (Eisner et al. 2000; Rona 2000). Asthma thus follows other conditions in exhibiting disparities in prevalence and severity by race/ethnicity. And, as with other medical conditions, biological meanings of race are used to account for these disparities in ways that affect the meaning of the disease. The search for the genetic predisposition to asthma among black populations is a search for explanations other than the economic or medical-access conditions shared by these populations.

Gene-environment research thereby gives new meaning to concepts of environment, disparities in asthma severity, and race (see, e.g., Barnes et al. 2001; Hall 2001; Xu et al. 2001; Ahmadi and Goldstein 2002; Fenech and Hall 2002; Morahan et al. 2002; Shapiro and Owen 2002). The Collaborative Study on Genetics of Asthma (CSGA), which has included research teams from Johns Hopkins University, University of Chicago, University of Maryland, University of Minnesota, and four other universities, has reported different asthma susceptibility loci among African American, Hispanic, and European American populations (Barnes et al. 2001; Shapiro and Owen 2002). The University of California at San Francisco (UCSF) Genetics of Asthma in Latin Americans Study focuses on Latino and African American asthmatics. In the case of response to asthma medications, a variant in a gene (β2 adrenergic receptor; β2 AR) thought to increase the severity of asthma and decrease the response to a type of medication (β2 agonists) is reported to exist in 37 percent of Caucasians in contrast to 49 percent of African Americans (Omenn and Motulsky 2003). A gene reported to influence response to another asthma medication (antileukotriene modifiers) has also been differentiated by racial group, and the genetic variations in CYP450-metabolizing genes that are differentiated by racial prevalence as discussed earlier affect response to asthma drugs too (Fenech and Hall 2002). These projects give shape to "race" and "asthma" and "environment" by formulating their interaction.

The Barbados Asthma Genetics Study

The Barbados Asthma Genetics Study is heralded by the team as having produced the largest database of asthmatics of African descent. The researchers have reported evidence of chromosome linkage with asthma and correlated this with African Americans, as part of the CSGA. Barbados is thereby brought into the genetics of asthma as a population considered representative of African Americans.

From the team's perspective, the perceived heterogeneity of the causes of asthma necessitates the focus on particular populations. The various possible environmental and genetic factors require studies attentive to the specificity of geographic area, climate, household behavior, and biological predispositions. Part of this specificity, for the research team, is a focus on race/ethnicity: the complexity of asthma—involving interactions of multiple genes and environmental factors—requires distinguishing effects such as racial/ethnic differentiation. As one article by the team puts it, "Because it is possible that different genes, as well as environmental exposures, influence asthma and asthma associated phenotypes in individuals of different ethnic backgrounds, three ethnic groups (African Americans, European Americans, and Hispanics) were ascertained in this study" (Xu et al. 2001: 1438). For the genetics team, this inclusion of race responds to a moral need to explain ethnic disparities of asthma.

The team members noted a similar prevalence, severity, and use of emergency departments for asthma by African Americans and Barbadians and contrasted these figures with those for Caucasians or the general U.S. population. In discussions, they considered ignoring race/ethnicity to allow research on Caucasians to be falsely representative of all populations. The group valued the genetics studies in Barbados partially as contrastive with other asthma genetics projects that do not include populations of African descent and thereby ignore diversity.[14] One member of the team described her research goals as focusing on the genetics of diseases that disproportionately affect minorities. Studies of genetic-environment interactions and race are thereby given a valence of morality as filling social and medical gaps: for the researchers, the genetics of asthma and race provides an important redress to a lack of research on populations who bear the larger burden of disease.

This interpretation gives new significance to genetic predisposition, environment, and race, through their interaction. As a gene-environment study, the project design was contrasted on one side with genetic susceptibility studies that fail to account for gene-environment interactions, such as the reciprocal influence of immune-response gene expression and allergen exposure. On the other side, the study design was posed against purely environmental studies that were considered more susceptible to factors that complicate results, such as age and socioeconomic status. As independent from these factors, genes are interpreted to be more stable and thereby more reliable in assigning causality. "Environment" is newly configured in this framing. The study has concluded that Barbadians have a high sensitivity to tropical mites, which is interpreted to be involved in asthma. The study's focus on a tropical country was contrasted with the focus of asthma research on developed countries: for the team, the Barbados research is a corrective to research that treats environments in developed countries as representative of the general asthmatic experience. The particularities of the Barbadian environment give a valence of social justice to the research as a step toward interventions particular to each environment. For example, a geneticist involved in the CSGA suggested that genetic predisposition might be part of the reaction to cockroach antigen that causes a high asthma prevalence and severity in urban areas such as Harlem (Lester et al.

2001). Here, race as a biological factor must morally be accounted for in studying the asthma experience among urban African Americans. In these extensions of gene-environment analyses, biological race interacts with social problems like urban housing disparities or conditions in developing countries.

But what occurs for the families, practitioners, officials, and researchers involved in these studies? How do these biomedical concepts get taken up in diverse ways, interacting with discourses of public health, family responsibility, ethnic identity, medical categories? The use and creation of biomedical categories occurs through such multiple interactions, producing unexpected meanings and practices. Biomedical categories, like goods in Boon's reading (1999: 299), "go crazy, or are already so 'foundationally.'"[15] They are created contradictorily and used compulsively. In this cultural life, excesses produce strange new objects, like the hyperdiagnostics of race, or, as we will see, estimates of asthma prevalence in a single population ranging from 18 percent to 80 percent. Attending to these moments of excess allows us to see researchers, practitioners, and patients as more than objects caught in institutional matrices. These individuals and communities interpret discursive formations such as the environment, race, and disease in diverse and often ambivalent ways that create their efficacy and allow them to be relevant to those involved.

Chapter 2

The Nation as Biomedical Site

Barbados as Genetic Site

Barbados is a center of international genetics-of-disease research. The various studies have been conducted by academic and industry research teams based in the United Kingdom and United States, including, in particular, teams from Johns Hopkins University and State University of New York (SUNY) Stony Brook. The current research includes searching for genetic propensity for cancers, asthma, acute lung injury, obstructive sleep apnea, asthma severity, and dengue fever (two studies, one American, one British). Previous genetic research in Barbados examined glaucoma. All of this research is premised on race. Biomedical research categorizes Caribbean populations as Afro-Caribbean, biologically equivalent to African American, in contrast to European, Caucasian, or other similar ethnic/racial distinctions. Researchers look for biological processes or genetic predispositions that characterize black populations. Studies have correlated Afro-Caribbean peoples as black with particular genetic predispositions for disease (Spencer et al. 2000; Kousta et al. 2001; Nemesure et al. 2003) or with a biological propensity for obesity, skin disease, and other conditions (Pomerleau et al. 1999; Dunwell and Rose 2003; Westermann et al. 2003).

Within this science of race in the Caribbean, Barbados is specifically chosen primarily because of the market mechanics of the state: the peculiar mix of a nationalized health care system and integration into global medical markets. The U.S. genetics team comes to Barbados for its robust medical facilities and records and the access to patient participants. The extensive international biomedical work relies on the Barbadian government: the projects are facilitated by the interaction of a U.S.- or U.K.-based research team and Barbadian physician/researchers usually through the Chronic Disease Research Centre, a division of the Barbados Ministry of Health (MOH). The MOH's system of disease classification and intervention provides records and, more importantly in the eyes of the genetics team, Barbadian physicians and nurses who facilitate the study—they collect data and recruit participants. The nationalized health care system is also significant for standardizing access to medicine and care, considered to make the population less heterogeneous than other groups and thereby more amenable to gene-environment research. Patients are understood to be particularly willing participants in the studies, which the researchers attribute to the high educational level and a value Bajans place on medical care. Mary Warner is a member of the Johns Hopkins team.[1] She indicated to me the significance of the educational levels for facilitating the study, noting, "They have a literacy rate higher than the U.S." As Carla Freeman (2000) has demonstrated, these qualities of social stability and educational levels have been significant in attracting international businesses to Barbados, and are used in trade rhetoric by both Barbadian officials and multinational companies. In the case of biomedicine, these features are used to present Barbadian citizens as good subjects for research and intervention.

The posing of Barbados as an ideal place for genetic research thereby includes a set of attributes that intimately link the state with the family: health care infrastructure and stability, patient acceptance of research, and educational levels interact to make a population advantageous to research. These characteristics are akin to other research advantages posited for other populations. In one discussion about why Barbadians are good candidates, a researcher explained to me that while they are not genetically isolated or homogeneous as are the Icelanders, this disadvantage was offset by the extraordinary health care system in place and the educational levels of Barbadians.

In this chapter, I explore such partnerships made between governments in resource-poor countries like Barbados and international bioscience and pharmaceutical institutions. I interviewed specialists, pediatricians, and family doctors in their offices in urban or rural private practices, in polyclinics, and at the hospital. I also interviewed pharmacists and nurses across Barbados. This analysis also draws from interviews and participant observation with Ministry of Health officials. National officials attempt to maximize public health by integrating international biomedical expertise and technologies into state medical facilities, physician training, and health education outreach. This global trade in medical research sites is producing unpredictable routines around public health and patient populations.

Private/Public Health

Barbados has considerable influence in the Caribbean, particularly in medical practices. Since gaining independence from England in 1966, the country has been comparatively politically and economically stable among the Caribbean countries. The national health care and education systems have resulted in a 13 percent poverty rate and a 98 percent literacy rate, according to the World Health Organization (WHO) and International Monetary Fund (IMF). Along with Jamaica, Barbados is a major source of medical knowledge for the English-speaking Caribbean. Physicians, researchers, and nurses conduct seminars in neighboring countries and act as consultants on formularies and medical infrastructure. This influence is largely premised on Barbados's National Drug Formulary.

Medicines on this Formulary are officially free to citizens younger than 16 or older than 64 who present their Barbadian identification and prescription to any state pharmacy (at the polyclinics and Queen Elizabeth Hospital [QEH]) or at participating private pharmacies (which includes almost all of them, to at least some degree (see chapter 6)). What this technically means is that a department of the MOH—the Barbados Drug Service—will reimburse pharmacies for a specified amount of a medication per month for each citizen with a valid prescription. Asthma is one of five conditions, epilepsy, hypertension, cancer, and diabetes being the others, for which medications are free to all citizens, with no age restrictions. This Formulary has made the multinational pharmaceutical industry integral to Barbadian health care. Barbados is now the center of the multinational pharmaceutical industry presence in the eastern English-speaking Caribbean. Representatives for the region are based in Barbados, and the country is the source of literature distribution, lecturers, and continuing medical education programs. This role of the industry extends beyond purveying medicines, as the national health care system relies on pharmaceutical companies for expertise and education about disease and care.

The Barbadian national health care system is composed of nine clinics distributed across the country and one large hospital (QEH) located in the relatively urban area called Bridgetown. The Accident and Emergency Department of the hospital receives 10,000 visits per year for asthma, accounting for 22 percent of its overall admissions. As the source of the most sophisticated technologies and care for poorer families, this department is utilized by patients for primary care (a practice also found in the United States). This department has an Asthma Bay, and patients that are identified as asthmatic are allowed immediate entry, unlike patients identified with other emergency conditions. The polyclinics receive considerably lower proportional levels of funding, resulting in much less use.

Multinational pharmaceutical companies are the primary source of medical literature and education programs for the hospital and polyclinics, and provide funding and international speakers for lectures on diseases and therapies. Janet Russel is an official in the MOH. During an interview at her office, she talked with me about the interaction of the government with the industry with respect to care: "What we try to do more at the Drug Service public lectures is get companies involved in sponsoring public events. We get good support—six hundred to a thousand people. Companies are intimately involved in care. We work with pharmaceutical reps to do CME [continuing medical education] with pharmacies." This mix of industry and government is consistent with Barbadian interactions of public and private sectors since the country became independent (Beckles 1990): unlike some other Caribbean countries, the Barbados government neither adopted a program of generalized state control of agriculture and other industries, nor embraced a strongly free market system, but instead blended both methods (e.g., the foundation for the economy, the sugar industry, was not taken over by the state but instead was taxed extremely heavily to fund public projects including QEH (Freeman 2000: 77)). The Formulary is an extension of this public care provided through the interaction of global markets and government facilitation. Such interaction is viewed ambivalently by many—including Janet herself—as both an important achievement and a capitulation to markets.

Contested Formulary

The National Drug Formulary is foundational to health intervention in Barbados, in terms of funding, techniques of intervention, and the discourse of state representatives. WHO used the list of medicines as a model, an accolade high-level medical officials often repeated to me. General practitioners and specialists prescribe almost exclusively from the Formulary. A private doctor I interviewed in his office in Bridgetown, Thomas Lancaster, explained the reason for this focus: "If I prescribe off the Formulary, patients don't get it anyway [because of the cost]."

This list is a source of deep disagreement in Barbados. Doctors, nurses, and pharmacists talked vividly and often angrily about the process of how medicines get on the Formulary, its relative efficacy, and its impact on Barbadian health. As a potent medical object, the Formulary is considered at once a significant tool of intervention, a symbol of the impact of multinational pharmaceutical companies, and a representation of the flaws in a commercialized public health care system. I first became interested in the Formulary when I heard pharmacists and doctors in interviews arguing that there were too many medications on it. Mitchell Baines, who runs an urban pharmacy, talked about this overabundance: "I agree [with a polyclinic doctor] that there are too many drugs available on the Formulary. There's not justification to have three or four of the same kind. That never was what the Formulary was intended for. It was meant to be: you tender, you win that tender, you get to sell the drug. Look at cholesterol: *seven* different drugs. All free." Doctors and pharmacists particularly emphasized an excess of patented pharmaceuticals. As I looked the list over, the number of brand-name medications did seem astounding. Vioxx and Bextra were there, and some medicines unavailable in the United States: Berotec, an asthma medication not approved by the FDA because of safety concerns, and Symbicort, a combination asthma inhaler not yet reviewed by the FDA, expected by analysts to become a blockbuster.[2] The availability of such a range of brand-name pharmaceuticals, in the eyes of many practitioners and pharmacists, reflected an undue government focus on the interests of the multinational pharmaceutical companies.

Two committees are involved in getting a drug placed on the Formulary. The Formulary Committee reviews applications to put a drug on the list, and those accepted go to the Tenders Committee, which approves a particular product. Both of these bodies are part of the Barbados Drug Service within the MOH. These Drug Service committees negotiate with the pharmaceutical industry to dramatically reduce the prices for the patented pharmaceuticals that are made available on the Formulary. Many of the physicians and most of the pharmacists I talked with argued that the industry had too much influence on the committees, as patented pharmaceuticals are purchased in place of generic drugs. Leon Castor is in his early thirties and runs a large urban pharmacy. During our conversation at this pharmacy, he talked with frustration and emotion about the medical care system. He is an outspoken critic of the government emphasis on medication access: "The Formulary for asthma is a wish list—Pulmicort [an inhaled steroid treatment for asthma] was out a year or two. There's no logical reason to have it on Formulary. It's lobbying." Leon's and similar accusations of drug industry influence on health care were not of corruption but of a legitimated pressure: these critics denounced the systematized integration of pharmaceutical industry agendas into state health interventions.

At times, this integration was posed as a simple market logic of exchange. Leon remarked, "It has been known, if a company has ten drugs on Formulary, they want a new one on, they will say, 'We'll give you ten of these at this price, if you will put this drug on Formulary.' Also the chief of the Tenders Committee has been known, once the Formulary Committee says, 'Not this drug,' to say, 'I don't care,' and put it on anyway." Leon is close to several high-ranking members in the industry and government and he spoke angrily about this basic exchange. He advocates a more "objective" medicine, and felt that acceptance of the multinational pharmaceutical companies' agenda damages public health as patients are given medications that are not therapeutically the best for them. He also echoed the majority of pharmacists in arguing that the cost of providing such excess medications precludes other types of intervention for these groups; Leon particularly focused on investment in better diagnostic technologies. For these health care practitioners, the market state logic has become irrational.

The object of this critique extended beyond the patented medications to include the biomedical research occurring in Barbados. This research is primarily conducted by multinational companies comparing the relative efficacy and safety of existing formulations and by British and U.S. academic institutions examining the genetics of diseases. For Leon, the pharmaceutical exchange system that produces both the research and the bias of the Formulary is part of a new approach to the patient:

> Companies will come and say they spend their money on research for treatment. They don't initiate research, it's not worth their while, it's a myth. They spend money on marketing, and they try to force the Barbados Drug Service to put their drug on Formulary. They say, "If you don't we will not support your seminars."...It's a bread basket for the drug companies. Market goals are shifting more to the patient.

Leon went on to argue that the research the pharmaceutical industry conducts in Barbados is about extending markets, not producing new medications. In his view, shared by most pharmacists and many doctors I talked with, the negotiations over pharmaceutical access and biomedical knowledge are interlinked forms of industry influence.

This critique resonates with arguments from social analyses on the impact of global markets on health. In the process of pharmaceuticalization described by the pharmacists and practitioners, health intervention is construed as access to pharmaceuticals, and other approaches to public health are marginalized (see Biehl 2004a on the context of AIDS intervention in Brazil). This practice is expanding in the current configurations of international trade under the Trade-Related Aspects of Intellectual Property Rights (TRIPS): government purchase of pharmaceuticals and accordance with patent and exclusivity laws are increasingly emphasized in this technique of health intervention in resource-poor countries (see Sell 2003). In Barbados, public health intervention relies on the hybrid of pharmaceutical company agendas and government national health care. The MOH relies on the pharmaceutical companies for health information and funding of outreach programs to physicians, teachers, and parents; the pharmaceutical companies rely on the Barbados Drug Service for inclusion of their products on a formulary that is influential throughout the English-speaking eastern Caribbean.

This configuration creates categorizations of Bajans as medical markets: for research, for pharmaceutical sales, and for Caribbean influence. But if the state is widely seen to be inordinately shaped by the interests of pharmaceutical companies in a market bureaucracy gone haywire, how do the public officials who enact this influence see their position? The government officials involved in these partnerships engage the market logics with their own reflections on the power of international companies on medical policy and government responsibility for public health. In order to follow these reflections, I turned to the Formulary and Tenders committees themselves. The focus on pharmaceutical access in contrast to, for example, toxic waste disposal legislation is a particular kind of market (ir)rationality, one that provoked anger, resistance, pride, and other meanings of nationalism among the very state representatives who facilitate it. The practitioners of pharmaceuticalization thereby critique the process of pharmaceuticalization in ways that reveal the unstable integration of global markets into state agendas.

State Oppositions

Membership in the Formulary and Tenders committees changes, but generally it includes MOH officials, pharmacy trade group representatives, pharmacists, and medical specialists from QEH, polyclinics, and private practice. I attended a Formulary Committee meeting, and interviewed several members of both committees in their offices at the MOH or in polyclinics, the hospital, pharmacies, or private practices, as well as during various interactions at medical meetings. In these conversations, the government officials involved in bringing the pharmaceutical industry into the public health system assessed this process as problematic. Members of the Drug Service committees (Formulary and Tenders) described an exchange relationship between the major pharmaceutical companies and the state: a trade fraught with social and material debt, antagonism and affinities. At times, a basic exchange system was presented in which companies threaten to end educational programs unless a particular drug is approved to go on the Formulary. But, as in the case of Michael Oldani's account of sales representatives and physicians in the United States (2004), this level of explicit market trade was rare. Instead, in Barbados a general move toward generic drugs, encouraged by the Pan American Health Organization, is effectively countered by pressures from the pharmaceutical industry. This general trend toward the use of brand-name drugs over generic ones was more subtle than trade of a particular drug on formulary for a particular program: the patented pharmaceutical becomes a social good through the reciprocal representations of care and markets by government officials and industry representatives.

These officials lamented the influence of the pharmaceutical industry on Barbadian health, sometimes angrily, sometimes dispiritedly. Members of the Drug Service committees talked about physicians writing letters to the committee promoting a medication that they had barely used, because the pharmaceutical company provided incentives for the physicians. They also implicated other Committee members as being overly influenced by particular companies, and each committee made similar accusations about the other. In general, there was a sentiment of constant pressure from the pharmaceutical companies; as one member put it, "It's like holding back the horses."

But this criticism of a barely controlled and eroding force occurred alongside the view that the industry is necessary to optimize care. A trade was considered critical to obtaining needed medical knowledge: the excess of patented pharmaceuticals on the Formulary was an acceptable exchange for the educational programs offered by the multinationals. Janet, the MOH official who talked about the pharmaceutical industry earlier, is a Drug Service Committee member. She explained this logic of mutual agreement between the government and multinationals to me: "They provide lots of education programs to the public which you do not find with the generics. That's why we need to coexist. We couldn't have optimal care without the education arm, and so we need to work jointly together for care."

As discussed, the education is extensive. Others echoed the sense that the multinationals were the only source of needed education, as Drug Service committee member Audrey Keyes explained to me, "The problem is that you can't get it from the generic companies. So that's the phenomenon you have to deal with. You can call Glaxo or AstraZeneca. But who would you call about the generic?" This level of industry involvement is often posed as a gift offered to the state. Representatives of multinational companies, and some government officials, depict the literature and funding as favors, an act of charity offered to the government's public health system. The reciprocal for this gift is more representation of patented drugs over generics on the Formulary.

The singular and intense pressures the multinationals exert were here posited as needed to maximize care. Janet's concept of needing to "coexist" interestingly implied an antagonism between the state and the industry. Optimization occurs only if the two recognize a need for each other despite divergent goals. A general practitioner, Gregory West, expressed this binary thus: "Well, they are in business in the making of money, so they're looking for a return. You have to have a balance."

The pharmaceutical multinational industry acts in these accounts as both a part of state intervention and a difficult to contain force influencing the state.[3] State medical care was posed as a product of the multinational-government relationship, obviating any easy distinction between global and local, or state and industry. For another Drug Service committee member, Silas James, the dissolution of this mix would result in a patient without an effective public health care system: "In my opinion, the government cannot continue to operate the system as we are doing it. At some point the companies are going to say we aren't going to do this anymore [i.e., offer education, reduce prices]. And who is going to suffer? The patient."

In this balance or coexistence, the counterweight to the industry's zealous market practices is the state acting as vigilant overseer of the pharmaceutical industry. The government thereby places itself in a kind of opposition-through-attention to the pharmaceutical industry's singular interest in selling products. Being aware of its interests becomes the accepted means of weathering the dangers. The antagonism implied by Janet toward the industry was common among the Drug Service committee members. The market practices involved in getting a drug to be considered by the committees were raised as a subject of concern, and at times, an object of scorn. This view of expert knowledge as deeply tied to market interests resulted in a positioning of the Formulary Committee as a resistance to such influence.

The posing of the Drug Service committees as in conflict with the industry created heated disputes over accusations of influence by the industry. In a conversation between Drug Service committee members, one remarked that the Tenders Committee had approved drugs that the Formulary Committee never evaluated. A case was brought up of a drug that was turned down by the Formulary Committee but then put on the Formulary by the Tenders Committee—"backdoored," as the member put it. These accusations revealed frustration and resignation at a perceived compromise of government autonomy caused by the insidious pressure of multinationals. Among the medical officials a vigilance is seen as needing to be tempered with affinity, with cooperation and use, in order to help the patient.

Medical Market Schismogenics

This ambivalent relationship to the multinational firms relied on the postcolonial government's vulnerable position in a global economy. Having access to brand-name pharmaceuticals was considered a highly precarious position for Barbados. As Janet put it, "Supply in brands or generics can stop for any reason: batch failure, unavailability of raw materials, sometimes worldwide. Or they just decide to pull that particular line, they decide they're no longer going to use it in developed countries, so we don't get it anymore. We are a developing country—we are just a drop in the bucket." Another Drug Service committee member, Vincent Kent, talked about an event reflecting this position: "When Glaxo merged with SmithKline in '99 or 2000, they forgot about the Caribbean! For a *year!* No drugs at all for over a year! None. Because of administrative oversight. Glaxo thought SmithKline would do it and SmithKline thought Glaxo would. So when Glaxo tries to take this benefactor stature, I remind them." As Vincent denounced the gift-giving status of the multinationals, he emphasized the vulnerability of being a small and relatively poor country/market. This position makes Barbados at the mercy of the temperamental global market changes, in his and others' view.

A Barbados Drug Service representative talked with me about these difficulties of being a small purchaser: "Some drug companies won't sell under a given amount, the order has to be large enough. So the BDS has trouble with rare drugs needed, where they don't have enough of an order." Silas commented, "The concern I have about it is that the globalization in markets and all the conglomeration of companies means that the problem's going to get worse. Bigger companies are taking over smaller companies and then they can say we won't supply that any more." John Lyndon is the head of a major distributor of pharmaceuticals in the eastern Caribbean, based in Barbados. He works closely with the MOH in designing medication access in Barbados. In an interview in his office, he talked about the significance of global economic changes on the pharmaceutical markets for medical care in the Caribbean:

> More and more multinationals are looking at markets. They don't even give you a guaranteed quantity. They give you an *estimated* quantity. I have one I represent, they say we're not going to stock anything in their regional warehouse that is not selling more than $250,000. So suddenly, I can't get it. Or they'll say, "We are no longer going to sell that product in the Caribbean." Suddenly, no support, no samples, and they're not going to stock it in their wholesale warehouses. They say, "Feel free to buy from our warehouse in London." But it will cost more, sometimes *six times* more, and we will have a contract that says we have to buy from that wholesaler. So now we have to go to them in Miami or wherever and ask if we can. So I have to say to them in Miami, "Can I buy from someone else?" They say, "Yes, but you have to buy from wholesalers," so the price goes up.

John works within this instability by anticipating responses and fluctuations in supplies. This volatility is especially heightened as the industry centralizes through corporate acquisitions. The purchase of smaller companies by multinational firms leads to variable availability of the medications they produce. He told me a story of four acquisitions leading to a company owning a product he supplied to the Barbados Drug Service. He continued:

> Barbados accounted for 87 percent of sales in [the product] in the Caribbean. But even at 87 percent, as you can imagine, it was not of interest to the fifth largest drug company in the world. So they decided, we are no longer selling it. So then I have to get it from England. But the cost there is 6.5 times the cost of it in the Caribbean.

Such centralization in the global market of pharmaceuticals affects the daily Formulary operations, according to Silas:

> There is the issue of doctors being manipulated by the big companies. For example, one company last week, they asked us about a product they tendered. I asked, "Are there any tests that have been done?" No. "Well, are there any doctors using the product?" They said one doctor. I said, "You can't be serious." But then what will happen is you will get a letter from the doctor

saying it's good. That has been happening *increasingly,* because, as the market shrinks to maybe five big companies, the competition is going to get more intense.

For Silas, as for Janet and Vincent, understanding the global market is considered crucial to the practice of the state in extending public health care through pharmaceutical access. The Drug Service committee members see the Barbadian state as needing to respond to this capricious system in order to optimize health.

In this approach, measuring the trends and effects of international institutions, such as the multinational corporations, the World Trade Organization, the World Bank, and IMF structural adjustment programs, becomes central to public health for small, resource-poor countries like Barbados.[4] Governments focus on anticipating and interpreting the motives, intentions, and retaliations of such transnational institutions.

This sociality of expectations and implied responses occurs outside of the formal regulations and provisions of trade agreements. Vincent told me a story that exemplified such policy based on anticipation. In recent years, AIDS has dramatically increased in Barbados. In the late 1990s, the MOH looked for ways to purchase antiretroviral agents. After a dispute within the MOH over the route to obtaining cheaper medication, a decision was made to work with the World Bank to get access, rather than go against multinational interests by purchasing pharmaceuticals from Indian companies. Vincent expressed his frustration with this process. According to him, this negotiation led to a result still weaker than what would have been achieved otherwise: "Three and a half years with the World Bank, and the result is a preference price for AIDS drugs that we would have got anyway. Over the last five years, with the World Bank, we made an agreement— it took three years, and lowered the price to something that we still can get a price at cheaper in Brazil or India." Here, despite TRIPS provisions that allow the Barbadian government to purchase the Indian drugs, the government, anticipating retaliation from the multinational pharmaceutical industry, elected to work with the World Bank. Vincent's exasperation with this process reflects the deep ambivalence state members felt toward this informal exchange in guesswork and pressures.

Analysis of the vagaries of the global market extended to the minutiae of drugs approved and integrated into the Barbadian health care system. For example, two Drug Service committee members discussed an antibiotic: the pediatric department of QEH was using large tubes of the antibiotic to administer small amounts in the absence of more suitable smaller tubes. The following discussion occurred between the two members:

LINDA: Erythromycin, why is it not available? We are using 5-gram tubes!

SHIRLEY: It's cheaper for us to use the 5-gram tubes, and throw it away.

ANOTHER DOCTOR: Sometimes it's not being thrown away, it's being given to the parents.

SHIRLEY: So I think the emphasis should be on hospital staff to throw it away.

LINDA: Why doesn't the committee try to get smaller amounts?

SHIRLEY: We tried, we just didn't succeed.

Here, understanding and working with the mercurial global market was considered critical to providing care. The informal economy of harmful antibiotic consumption that was thereby produced is then made the responsibility of individual physicians, instead of a systematic practice.

These reciprocal interactions comprise a market schismogenesis, to use Gregory Bateson's term (1958): government and pharmaceutical industry representatives interact in a complementary, reciprocal process, each accentuating his or her stance in relation to the other's reaction. These schismogenics were particularly visible with regard to the pharmaceutical patent. Barbados has yet to break patents through compulsory licensing or importing of generic drugs. In the absence of a local granting of patents, the Barbadian government uses a system of negotiation in which multinational pharmaceutical companies argue that patents in effect in other countries (primarily the United States and United Kingdom) are in effect in Barbados. As Janet put it, "We just relied on the overseas, we will piggyback on them, meaning the patent lasts as long as that country's." Silas emphasized the capriciousness of this practice, arguing that it gives undue power to the multinational representative to choose which country represents the overseas registration. Vincent spoke angrily about the perceived disingenuousness involved, referring to a particular medicine: "[It] was available eighteen months before in Europe than in the U.S. Therefore, the American company, for four or five years past their patent, they tried to convince us that it was still patented because patented in another country." The representation of international trade was here posed as a space for ethics. For Vincent, Barbados, a country signatory to TRIPS, could make use of compulsory licensing provisions by which pharmaceuticals could be obtained cheaper through local manufacturing or importation. He continued,

"We honor patents as a favor. If companies continue to be so unethical, why should we?"

When pharmaceutical multinationals threatened to withdraw certain medications or programs, the government responded by threatening to make use of compulsory licensing provisions. The Barbados attorney general has argued that only drug patents that have been filed in Barbados are valid. Since no multinational firm had at the time filed such a patent, all of the brand-name drugs would be off patent if this law were enforced. But the state members I spoke with largely considered this an empty threat. However, it has been used at times to justify removal of particular drugs from the Formulary, according to some members. Silas told such a story: "I will let you in on a secret. In June of last year we had a meeting with the attorney general. All of these suppliers were there. So when I arrived, they wanted to look at the laws covering the patents. Merck owned Pepcid, and Pepcid was kicked off in [favor of a producer] in India. The rep made a fuss about it." Silas drew attention to such myriad negotiations around global markets by which the Formulary policy is made.

Such a sociality extends beyond pharmaceuticals. The shift to tourism as the primary industry has resulted in a constant assessment of public image by state representatives. Analysis of the international market is the basis for environmental interventions, as I found in interviews with government officials responsible for the regulation of pesticides and industrial chemicals. One official involved in pesticide control remarked, "[We're] moving more toward shifting from use of pesticides, especially now with the global shift, so if we are to export to these markets, we must be below the levels. And with the tourists especially from Europe and the U.S. Take Barbados—if one tourist came down sick, it wipes out the tourism industry."[5] Regulations rely on a hyperawareness of the country's position within the global market. Because of its reliance on tourism, foreign aid, and pharmaceutical access, the government attends to how Barbados is represented in the global economy when making public health, toxic waste, and pesticide policy.

These interpretations and anticipations of responses from multinational institutions are often overlooked in the emphasis on trade agreements and policies. Government representatives viewed positions taken by multinational pharmaceutical subsidiaries in Barbados to be rhetorical moves: the threats to withdraw educational programs or a needed drug were countermoves to calls for a shift to generic drugs by the minister of health. The accusations by Tenders and Formulary committee members of mutual influence were themselves reactions born out of the value and difficulties of resisting such pressures, and the ambivalence of wanting and denouncing the impact of pharmaceutical companies. If local subsidiaries can convince the MOH that GlaxoSmithKline will respond by withdrawing a drug, or that new medicines are on the verge of making another one obsolete, then policy can be effected. These guesses, bluffs, and implicit warnings make regulatory documents like TRIPS into social objects: the explicit provisions for poor countries can be undermined by implicit representation and implied reprisals. The government enacts a medical policy around patented pharmaceuticals through these global economic schismogenics— market responses and consequences guessed at or heard in interactions between government officials and multinational representatives.

Barbados as Metropole

As is clear from this discussion, the most common view of Barbados was a country at the mercy of the global economy. As Silas put it:

> I am aware that the minister of health now wants to move as much as possible to generic. But the bigger companies are buying up the generic. They'll buy the generic company for one drug the generic company makes, and not for the others. So it's nothing for Pfizer to buy a generic for one drug, and the others are ended. So we are at the mercy of the marketplace. We can't make any demands to pay at a preferential price. We are so small.

U.S. and European multinationals exemplified political economic power relations in these accounts. The history of colonialism was implicated by this discourse in complex ways. At times global capitalism was posed as reproducing the power relations of colonial hierarchies: government officials and medical practitioners noted the unidirectional flow of expertise, pollutants, and poor-nutrition food from the United States and United Kingdom to Barbados. Additionally, many Barbadians expressed anger about Barbados's former reliance on sugar production, which colonialism created: public officials, medical personnel, and others talked with resentment about this dependence on a single market and the economic impact of the decline in the international sugar market. The consequent focus on tourism was similarly criticized as a precarious industry that makes Barbados reliant on the wealthier countries. This shift was associated with the World Bank, which was associated with the United States and United Kingdom, and these countries were consequently criticized, particularly with the decline in tourism following the September 11th attacks on the United States. But in other contexts, many Barbadians categorized the United States as non-British, and associated American values with anticolonialism. For example, U.S. business models were talked about as flexible and allowing enterprising individuals to succeed, in contrast to British hierarchies. Teenagers and young adults particularly expressed identification with the United States in opposition to England and colonialism, through clothing and music styles (see Gilroy 1993b). These young people increasingly were choosing menial jobs with international businesses in an explicit rejection of jobs on sugar plantations, which were considered representative of England's history of power over Barbados.[6] These evaluations by Bajans I met included officials who at times positioned multinationals with the United States as not a British hierarchy, which could be utilized to good effect; at other times they positioned the multinationals as one of the many transnational institutions that make Barbados beholden to global political economics.

But at times public officials reversed this interpretation of Barbados as caught within global political forces. When they talked about the country's position in the region, a very different representation emerged in which influence and expertise extended outward. In this context, Barbados is considered a metropole in the eastern Caribbean in terms of modernization, integration into the global economy, and medicine.

The flow of medical expertise and medicines from Barbados to the eastern Caribbean reflects this position. As mentioned, the pharmaceutical industry for the English-speaking eastern Caribbean is centered in Barbados, and the sales representatives I spoke with would travel to market pharmaceuticals to the other Caribbean islands from their homes and offices in Barbados. The amount of sales in Barbados reflects this centralization: as one pharmaceutical sales representative told me, "We [the company] sell more [β2 agonists] here than in Trinidad." Leon talked about the movement of medicines and medical information: "Trinidad, the eastern Caribbean, the reps start here, and they will go over there, so a lot of the education comes from here. It's not really home grown. Barbados is the center for this part of the Caribbean, so drug companies will bring a doctor here." Barbadian specialists are paid to consult and conduct educational programs for government health care in other countries. The pharmaceutical industry facilitates this travel, funding Caribbean health organizations that bring national experts from Barbados to Trinidad and other countries. This influence also extends to the Organization of Eastern Caribbean States (OECS), the economic and political institution that represents the eastern English-speaking Caribbean countries excluding Barbados. OECS operates with a centralized system for drug distribution, for which the Barbadian

MOH is a consultant. Supplier John talked about the relationship between Barbados and the eastern Caribbean through this drug service:

> The [drug service] applies only in the government clinic. It does not apply to the private sector, only in government hospitals. Each island orders individually. But the order goes to a central ordering section in St. Lucia. They do try to make four big purchases a year.... Their economies are not as strong as Barbados is. And multinational companies have not given the same level of support as in Barbados.

Barbados is thus a center for care, education, and pharmaceuticalization in the eastern Caribbean from the perspectives of both industry and government officials. Drug Service committee member Janet talked with me about this positioning: "We act as a resource—other countries pattern their services after ours. We have done several consultancies, in Guyana, St. Vincent, Trinidad."

The pride evident in such statements is a crucial aspect of the course of Barbadian public health policy. Janet's posing of the pharmaceutical industry as necessary but antagonistic to the state occurred alongside her pride in the intervention created through their involvement. She continued, "The education, you don't get this on other islands." I found a similar conflicted perspective in discussions about pharmaceutical industry ethics. The condemnation directed at the power of the multinational pharmaceutical companies also allowed them to be benefactors: posed as unethical in distribution or marketing practices, companies have the potential of being good; the dearth in morality of their practices posits a corollary possibility of an excess of moral practices. A professor at the University of the West Indies in Barbados offered such an account, after talking about the lack of research on vaccines by the pharmaceutical industry:

> My student at London College became the CEO of Glaxo Wellcome. He was a ruthless man. That group that year was very competitive. I tried to get some funding for some research I was doing here. The letter finally reached him and they had me come out to see him—lunch and so forth. Anyway, he told me we don't really fund research, and he cut me a check for twenty thousand. Pounds, not dollars.

Here, the frustration with the perceived influence of multinationals was inextricable from the attempts to gain from that influence in order to accomplish something good. (And from the professor's smile at my expression of surprise about the amount of money, I had the sense that he was pleased to convey his own level of influence in this process.) Such moments of simultaneous critique, pride, and want are foundational to evaluations and uses of pharmaceutical company practices for the postcolonial country.

These moments of vexation, irony, debt, are integral to the exchange systems that make use of international markets. Representations of Barbados within the Caribbean community, as a former colony, as a market, as a global economic or biomedical resource, are all used by government officials in understanding and creating pharmaceuticalization. Representing the market becomes a part of its operations, and reflexively. As Drug Service committee member Vincent put it, "The Formulary is a crock. We try to create competition where there wouldn't be competition because we are so small." In this framing, the Formulary is a device for Barbados to present itself as a market: through the Formulary, which is influential in the Caribbean, the government represents Barbados, thereby effecting a public health care system based on access to pharmaceuticals. Vincent treats the Formulary as a representation, a positioning tool in the attempt to make use of the international trade in pharmaceuticals.

Barbados's government-industry practice toward public health care intervention is thus not simply a facilitation of the global market in pharmaceuticals. This state approach relies on seeing Barbados as a leader in the Caribbean (e.g., as non-Trinidadian) and as having an autonomous public system (e.g., not a British colony). Government officials generate an identity as being at the forefront of biomedicine and thereby utilizing and maximizing the global economy that is elsewhere posed as an overwhelming political economic force. This national identity based on harnessing the global economy was also evident in state uses of biomedical research, as I explore later. The industry-government hybrid derives from this peculiar combination of anger and pride at multinational influence on the state. Like other postcolonial governments, Barbados enacts a kind of frustrated marketization: the facilitation-with-denunciation of the market into resource-poor public health care and economic systems.

Facilitating and Contesting the Medical Market

In Barbados, this sociality of regulation and marketization makes ambivalence foundational to the use of global medical markets. Vincent poses a model of capitalism in which economic interests are intrinsic and naturalized (outside human agency), pathological and irrational in its pursuit of profit, with regulation as the rational counter, the state intervention. This incorporates *and implicates* nationalism, a fetishized law as intervention, an ethics of global capitalism, and a binary of state versus multinational industry. Institutions such as the state, multinational companies, and the medical care system exist and thrive through conflicting and contradictory practices. The critical point is that the representations of ethics, of market irrationalities, and posing of global economic practices operate to facilitate these practices. Silas surprised me with a mix of pride and anger in telling a story about the sale of a medication to an American. The drug is sold in Barbados at a cheaper price than in the United States, but is also not placed under the same restrictions of safety and efficacy in manufacturing as imports to the United States are:

> An example of this happened with Zantac. Zantac was made available at a price that was almost 90 percent less than in the U.S. So you would have patients who would come here on a cruise liner, they would say, "How did you get it at that price?" Of course they are not aware that they are coming from Guatemala or Panama because GSK has a facility there.

In this story, Silas, the staunch critic of the perceived vagaries of the global economy for a small resource-poor country, lauded the victory of the availability of a drug at a cheaper price than in that symbol of wealth, the United States. By locating the production of these drugs in Guatemala or Panama, he was simultaneously angrily reflecting on the perceived variability of regulation by which his country is exposed to potentially unsafe medications not found in the United States. Public health is marketized culturally, as it is created and critiqued by its practitioners.

Silas talked further about the distinctions between the United States and Barbados, turning to the issue of being a small market:

> Then there's the other side where a company will say, "The minimum amount you will have to buy is 250,000 bottles." So we will say, "We can't buy it from you." Do we go through a broker? That means a markup. How much do you need it? A decision has to be made in terms of *business,* not in terms of medicine or the patient. A business decision is made about whether or not it's economically viable.

Here, Silas embraced a neoliberal economic evaluation, but self-consciously. Recognizing some alternative approaches and expressing his criticism and acceptance are part of his political economic stance. During another interview, he talked about this ambivalence:

> I am also concerned about testing the product for its quality. Who is doing the testing on these products? On efficacy? So the people who are really suffering is the patients. People can say I want my Norvasc and they can pay for it....I have on one side the patient and on the other the profit margin. I am caught between two sides.

The Barbadian public health system is effected through such formulated quandaries. Some critique the reliance on pharmaceutical access to the exclusion of other kinds of health intervention—for example, pollution legislation or health education. As Drug Service committee member Audrey Keyes expressed her frustration and resignation to me, "Here in Barbados, health care is health care, environment is environment, and education is education. We don't bring them together." The configuration of pharmaceutical multinationals and government operates in often surprising ways, allowing moments of resistance to be moments of facilitation.

These contradictions not only enable the global economy but also open up alternatives. Vincent in private discussions offered a significantly different view of public health. He criticized current biomedical techniques, arguing for a public health model in which the state would intervene at the family level through education of bodily health, sports, school programs, and information outreach on nutrition. This model diverged from his work as a Drug Service committee member in which the focus was on pharmaceutical intervention on individualized citizens. The simultaneous harboring of these mutually inconsistent approaches allows Vincent's enactment of the global market into policy.

In this exchange system, U.S. and British models of regulation and transparency become forms of intervention. To the Barbadian officials, these were the tools of reaction, allowing rejection of the pharmaceutical market practices to have effect. Silas talked with moral pride about his own defiance:

> The Director tried to tell the committee she would put a particular drug on. Reid, Jameson and myself, we are the three rebels. We will leave the room, you have to maintain your transparency. But then we have had cases of the Tenders Committee telling the Formulary Committee what drug they expect to be placed on the Formulary—the director has.

The models of transparency and British regulation for Silas became the legitimized techniques of resisting the flood of multinational interests. Such practices make pharmaceuticalization operate in convoluted and unexpected ways. The Formulary regulatory system that the pharmaceutical executives berated was what enabled them to use Barbados as a center of influence over the eastern Caribbean. The posing of pharmaceutical industry practices as gifts makes it possible to deny them as unethical. These schismogenics make cultures of global markets like pharmaceuticalization operate with unexpected twists and turns.

Situating Biomedical Research in the State

This mix of desire and denunciation also comprises the government's engagement with the several international biomedical research projects occurring in Barbados, including the Johns Hopkins genetics studies. As officials attract and evaluate such research, they draw on Barbados's political economic position in the Caribbean, a valued internationalism, and the population as needing such market interventions. Speaking of the various biomedical projects occurring, a former head of one of the highest government offices told me, "I have always advocated [international research]. If we are going to become a knowledge-based society, we need to have research. Barbados is a natural place for research: people are generally cooperative, it's a small society, it's a closed society, so you can get a grip on it." This official placed Barbados in the biomedical market system both as a population with characteristics that make it an ideal site for international research, and as requiring interaction with the market to remain a leader in medicine.

The government poses its population as conducive to international genetics research and the research as necessary to the population. At a public lecture in November of 2003, the Barbadian minister of health introduced Ian Wilmut, the geneticist who led the team that cloned Dolly. The minister talked about the several genetic studies occurring in Barbados, and the hope for gene therapy, discussing the international work on cancer and glaucoma as the future of biomedicine. These genetic projects were cast as essential to medical policy, owing to the increasing significance of genetics in international medical practice. The minister positioned Barbados as needing to take part in these developments: "The possibilities are limitless....We must not be left behind." Government rhetorics thereby link Barbadian health and medical care to the country's value as a site of international biomedical research.

The significance of this internationalism was emphasized in an interview I conducted with Edward Wright, a Barbadian government researcher involved in almost all of the international biomedical research occurring in Barbados. Detailing the history of medical research in Barbados, he focused on the studies that extended beyond Barbados: "No significant major research reaching the international scene occurred until early cardiovascular work...in the 1970s." In the subsequent discussion of the many foreign-based projects, the international significance was considered critical: "The Barbados Eye Studies received four consecutive NIH grants and led to the publication of more than thirty reviewed papers." He spoke with fervor of the various projects: the International Study on Hypertension in Blacks; the Barbados Asthma Genetics Study; the Cancer Study, also funded by the NIH ("I believe this is the only NIH-funded project with a non-American P.I. [principal investigator]"); two Wellcome Trust projects; and European Union funding of HIV research. The political connections with the United States confer a cosmopolitan biomedical status.

This embrace of global biomedicine plays into long Caribbean traditions of political positioning as "international." Edward discussed competition with Jamaica: "Jamaica is far in advance in terms of medical research activity...several decades ahead of Barbados." However, according to Edward, Barbados maintained its position as the center for biomedicine in the eastern Caribbean: "People come from the OECS to Barbados for medical treatment." He spoke with pride about the fact that "thirty papers from Barbados are presented every year at the Caribbean conference on medicine." Like the public officials, he also positioned this research as necessary to the health of the population: "Research is not only fundamental to medical training, but fundamental to health."

As with the National Drug Formulary, this use of international biomedicine generates deep ambivalence. Like Edward, many state members talked with pride about the various studies, and linked them to pharmaceutical industry research on the use and efficacy of types of medications as expanding health knowledge. Others criticized the motives and program of the research. Silas talked about the glaucoma part of the eye study: "These funding agencies have a certain amount of time, then they cut it off." He criticized such arbitrariness as due to financial interests. Silas advocates instead research on cost-effectiveness of medical care: "The hospital needs a research department to look at the cost of management within the hospital—pharmacist management." Such social approaches were often explicitly contrasted with the pharmaceutical comparisons and lab studies that are commonly talked about at local meetings and lectures.

These are the practices by which biomedical research, including the asthma study, is simultaneously effected and critiqued through concepts of nationalism, internationalism, and global markets. Like the pharmaceuticals on the Formulary, biomedical research is positioned ambivalently, facilitated into the health care system in Barbados by state members who elsewhere symbolically undermine such approaches. Drug Service Committee member Audrey offered such a conflicted account:

> Because I see the patient every *month* or more, I know what they're taking, I know if they're compliant. I talk to them. The doctor will go months without seeing them. I am the one who tells them, "Oh, you are diabetic. You should be taking this." One woman called me, she is coughing, and I find out she's taking an ACE inhibitor. Well, one of the side effects is dry cough. And she thought it was to do with her illness! So we are the ones who know about the patient.

Audrey considered the lack of discussion of side effects critical to patients' nonadherence to treatment. She advocated intervention by the pharmaceutical industry through education and provision of simplified medications to deal with this socially produced problem. She valued the simplicity of inhalers such as Symbicort as a response to the inadequate information on medical care. But she also harshly criticized the focus of research in Barbados on the efficacy of medications and biomedical techniques: "We need to address the *social* aspect. I believe in *social* pharmacy. In knowing what the cultural parts of medicine are. You've been to the Chronic Research Centre? They don't have any research on the *social*. None." Thus one Drug Service committee member criticized the medical care system as causing nonadherence and biomedical research as ignoring the social, while she supported the pharmaceutical as intervention on this dearth. Such paradoxical perspectives on market-driven medicine, state responsibility, and the limits of biomedicine are part of global market schismogenics that both facilitate and open alternatives to the administration of the pharmaceutical as preventive medicine and international biomedical research as a form of care.

Chapter 3

Asthma Variations

Asthma in Barbados has only recently taken shape as a diagnostic category through the focused attention of the pharmaceutical industry, biomedical research, and the state. This (re)categorization has drawn on the multiple techniques and deep disagreements that have characterized American and British medical meanings of "asthma." Before turning to the ways Barbados reflects and enhances this contestation, I here pause to explore this history of variation.

Early Symptoms and the Asthmatic Nervous System

At the end of the seventeenth century, asthma took shape as particular to a group, the asthmatics, as opposed to a generalized condition, in the work of Sir John Floyer (1698).[1] To Floyer, blood circulation was central to asthma, as was common with the humoral understanding of health and illness. Asthma was composed of a congeries of symptoms: wheezing, fever, intermitting pulse, and bronchial constriction.[2] Floyer listed numerous causes, including inflammatory tumor, abscess, coagulation of blood in the vessels, and adhesion of the lungs to the diaphragm, among others. Through his humoral interpretation, Floyer also considered excess consumption to cause attacks: "The Blood of Asthmatic is very subject to Effervescences; and whatsoever produces that, occasions the Fits; as great Heat or Cold, violent Motions of the Body or Mind, and Excess in Eating and Drinking, or Venereal Pleasures" (37). The idea that excess food was a cause of asthma attacks linked the stomach to the condition: "this fulness of the Stomach is the first sign of the ensuing Fit" (37).

In the nineteenth century, asthma as a grouping of experiences and causes transformed into a disease with a single locus. In 1860, Henry Hyde Salter offered a considerably different vision of asthma in his equally influential text. Salter and Floyer continue to be cited today as founders of modern perspectives on asthma. In the transition from Floyer of 1698 to Salter of 1860, the significance of lungs, diet, blood, and emotions to asthma changed. Where Floyer saw a collection of symptoms, Salter saw a condition defined by not leaving a physical mark, as historian Carla Keirns notes (2004). Salter wrote:

> The disease shows no cause, and has left no trace, either in the respiratory or circulatory systems—in fact no trace anywhere. Where, then, shall we locate it? What is its starting-point? We may, I think, lay it down as a rule, that all those diseases that leave no organic trace of their existence produce their symptoms through the nervous system. (1860: 30)

Michel Foucault's work points toward the radical break of this illness interpretation with Floyer's. According to Foucault (1994b.: 122), in the nineteenth century "the medicine of symptoms will gradually recede, until it finally disappears before the medicine of organs, sites, causes, before a clinic wholly ordered in accordance with a pathological anatomy." The question of where to locate the disease, its starting point, for Foucault, would not have been asked in the time of Floyer.[3] This question posits a mapping of the disease in the body, by which the disease's identity is constituted in a single site. Such identification contrasts with Floyer's collection of symptoms by which asthma is known. In Floyer's account, it remained unclear whether blood circulation caused rare respiration, or the reverse. Such a lack of spatial causality was no longer possible in the mid-nineteenth century. Instead, Salter would identify the condition by locating its site: this locus was the nervous system.

This simplicity resulted in a restriction of asthma to one process: while factors that brought on asthma attacks and kinds of treatment continued to be heterogeneous, the disease was no longer variable, but instead found in a single mechanism. In contrast to Floyer's various characteristics defining asthma—wheeze, unusual blood circulation, fever, coldness of the extremities, and so on—Salter (1860: 39) offered the nerve reflex: "the phenomena of asthma are those of excito-motory or reflex action." He described what was meant by this definition of asthma:

> Whenever the peripheral application of a stimulus results in a muscular motion, we say that the phenomena are reflex. And so they are, universally. As far as our present knowledge goes, we believe that a stimulus applied to a sentient surface or organ must first be transmitted to a nervous centre by incident, and thence reflected by motor filaments, before it can affect the muscular tissue, and stimulate it to contraction. (39)

For Salter, these physiological muscle responses were inextricable from emotional and mental states. Asthmatics had a particularly "sensitive" nervous system, which included a volatile temperament and motor responses. This sensitivity was gendered: "An asthmatic nervous system is a mobile, sensitive nervous system, and certainly the female nervous system is more mobile and sensitive than the male" (109).

This nervous disposition had many causes, which could be used to categorize the type of asthma. One category, "intrinsic asthma," was that in which an "irritant is applied to the lungs themselves" (114). Intrinsic asthma included cases caused by fog, animal emanations, and "blood poisoning"— including beer, wine, and sweets (114). Salter considered food, drink, smoke, and allergens potential causes of asthma because each was "applied to the lungs." Of these, food was the most important:

> But one of the peculiarities of asthma is that it may be induced by stimuli applied to remote parts: in these cases the nervous circuit is much longer, and the phenomena of reflexion clearer and more conspicuous. Take, for example, that most common of all the varieties of asthma, what we may call *peptic asthma*, in which the induction or prevention of attacks is entirely controlled by the state of the digestive organs; in which an error in diet— the eating some [sic] particular thing, eating too early or late in the day—is sure to bring on an attack; while a certain dietetic abstention is as certain to be attended with immunity from the disease. Here the reflex character of the phenomena is clear, and the nervous circuit by which the reflexion is completed conspicuous and evident. (40)

The asthmatic nervous system connected the stomach, blood, lungs, and emotional and mental states. Asthma was thus a kind of physiological neurosis for Salter—a reflex arc linking food, emotional characteristics, and motor response—without the subsequent categorical distinctions between mental and physiological that would later be central to the disease concept.

Treating the Nervous System

With this asthmatic nervous system, treatment was altered. Salter took an interesting route distinguishing symptom from disease through their different treatments:

> The treatment of asthma, like that of all paroxysmal diseases, naturally divides itself into the treatment of the paroxysm and the treatment in the intervals of the paroxysms, and although the last is the real treatment of the disease, while the treatment of the paroxysm is merely the treatment of a symptom, yet the paroxysm being in asthma, potential though not essentially, the disease (for it is its sole manifestation, the only source of suffering and the cause of those organic changes in the heart and lungs by which alone asthma threatens life), its treatment holds the first place in the therapeutics of the affection. (1860: 161)

The symptom, no longer the identity of the disease, became the primary site of treatment. Now the physician would treat the disease as a nervous system disorder, but only in order to reduce the symptoms. Relaxing the nerves thereby became the central role of treatment: depressants and contra-stimulants were "a class of remedies that exercises the most singular and powerful influence over the asthmatic condition, greater and more immediate than any other that I know, except, perhaps, mental emotion" (164). These treatments again made mental state, emotional disposition, and physiological reflex inextricable: "No doubt they all act in the same way—by lowering innervation, depressing nervous vitality or irritability, or whatever we may call it, and enfeebling the contraction of the bronchial muscle, just as they weaken the heart's action" (164). As Keirns (2004) argues, drawing from Keith Wailoo, treatments not only reflect but also constitute definitions of diseases. Salter's treatments were based on his concept of the asthmatic nervous system, but they were also evidence in support of such a classification in his view:

> Again the *remedies* of asthma are such as appeal to the nervous system—as antispasmodics, sedatives, direct nervous depressants, &c; tobacco, for example, stromonium, antimony, chloroform. Perhaps the effect of chloroform is, of all remedies, the most striking, and at the same time the most illustrative

of the purely nervous nature of the affection—a few whiffs, and the asthma is gone; a dyspnoea that a few seconds before seemed to threaten life is replaced by a breathing calm and tranquil. Now, that it is the nervous system to which it appeals, it is impossible to help seeing in this the most conclusive proof that the systems are due to a nervous cause. (Salter 1860: 26)

For Salter, the emotional, mental, and physiological were inextricable in a temperamental asthmatic nervous system, and this was proved by the efficacy of treatments that acted on such a configuration.

Salter was not the first to use these treatments for asthma. He referred to the common use of these and similar treatments (e.g., coffee and opium). Similarly, his directions to avoid excess food were shared by medical practitioners who had written about asthma earlier (e.g., Bree 1797) and contemporarily (e.g., Thorowgood 1870). His reflex arc was a predominant view within the mid-nineteenth century and, through his and others' work, the inherent and inherited were joined exclusively in the neurosis type of asthma.

Measurement, Neuroses, and Allergies

In the second half of the nineteenth century, as Keirns (2004) demonstrates, technologies became more involved in the categorization of asthma. According to Keirns, the microscope was used to search for germs and pollens as causes. "Respirometers," instruments that measured exhalation, were also employed to mark the distinction between asthmatics and non-asthmatics (see Braun 2005). Other technologies were used diagnostically or for treatment—for example, the "pleximeter" (Kingscote 1899) and antiseptic inhalers (Keirns 2004). With these techniques, quantitative measurements gave shape to the asthmatic condition. But amid this instrumentalization, giving concrete specificity to the condition, asthma continued to be explicitly defined by contrast: as nervous because no pathological lesions were found or as allergic because no germ causes were found. The germ theory, in Keirns's analysis, resulted in asthma being distinguished from consumption: tuberculosis was a disease of germs and antiseptics; asthma by contrast was a disease of heredity and constitution. In this context, causes and treatments continued to be highly heterogeneous: treatments included sedatives, stimulants, depressants, change in locale, and diet restrictions (Keirns 2004). In the second half of the nineteenth century asthma was increasingly quantitatively measured while divergently defined through a vague use of diatheses; of nervous dispositions; of reactions to various emotional, mental, and physical stimuli.

Through the end of the nineteenth and in the early twentieth century, this plurality of causes of asthma produced competing definitions along disciplinary lines, as Keirns (2004) argues. In the United States, the divergence of immunology and psychoanalysis in categorizing and exploring the condition resulted in a split between the physiological and the emotional/mental. The physiological aspects of asthma were primarily defined by allergists in terms of immune response to pollens and other allergens. Psychoanalytic tools were used to account for the interaction of mental and emotional dispositions with this physical response. Psychosomatic approaches to asthma in the early 1900s examined the disease as either partially or entirely a neurosis. At times the diagnosis itself, and the consequent mother's attention to it, were interpreted as causative: "Practically the child lives and is brought up in an atmosphere of 'asthma.' The 'traumatic insult' which the disease originally produced is converted into a 'psychic trauma,' and every functional disturbance, however slight, is apt to react adversely upon respiration" (Berkart 1916: 23). In these readings of mental and emotional conflicts and disorders, the family became a kind of agentive force in asthma. One review from 1931 attributed asthma to children deliberately having attacks to achieve certain ends; imitation of the asthmatic parent; and overprotection from the parents (Bray 1931). The distinction introduced between psychoanalytic accounts of such emotional and mental states on the one hand, and immunologists' theories of physiological responses on the other, created the basis for removal of the former from asthma models. In the 1950s and 1960s, with the U.S. move away from psychoanalysis, asthma became a purely physiological process, defined as an allergic response by allergists and as a lung tissue response by pulmonary experts.

Treatment in the United States in the early twentieth century reflected these differing causes and disciplinary techniques: by the mid-1920s, adrenaline, then theophylline and ephedrine, allergy shots, and diet restrictions were all employed. Keirns (2004) argues that these treatments, like Salter's, were not simply reflective but instead constitutive of asthma definitions; adrenaline in particular was considered to delineate the disease. Increasingly in the early-twentieth-century United States, pharmaceutical intervention was used to define the disease.

Genetic Inheritance

As has been indicated, heredity was associated with asthma before 1900. Floyer (1698), who was himself asthmatic, wrote, "As my Asthma was not Hereditary from my Ancestors, so, I thank God, neither of my two Sons are inclined to it, who are now past the Age in which it seized me." In 1860, Salter wrote, "Is asthma hereditary? I think there can be no doubt that it is" (109). Heredity in these accounts was a vague and peripheral aspect of asthma: while a part of the condition, little interest or focus was placed on heredity. Salter wrote of this inheritance "sometimes it is direct, sometimes lateral; sometimes immediate, sometimes remote" (109). Salter divided "all cases of asthma" into two groups. One was composed of organic lesions of the bronchial tubes or some part connected to them. The second category of asthma by cause was more nebulous for Salter: "Cases in which any organic lesion is not only inappreciable but non-existent, in which the tendency to asthma is due to something from within, not from without, in which the essential cause of the disease is a congenital, and possibly inherited, idiosyncracy" (134). Salter's uncertain wording leaves what is inherited and how open to question. He continued, "I steer, therefore, a middle course between those who say that asthma always has at the root of it some organic disease within the chest, and those who deny that genuine spasmodic asthma ever depends on organic lung-disease and maintain that it is always a pure neurosis" (134). Salter distinguished asthma caused by lesions from asthma caused by "something from within," which was asthma as neurosis. The "possibly inherited" asthma of the nineteenth century was a neurosis, an unspecified tendency, distinguished from asthma caused by a physiological effect on the bronchia or surrounding tissue. In the twentieth century, inheritance would have the opposite association.

In the early twentieth century, the idea of Mendelian heredity (one among many on heredity) changed how diseases were analyzed.[4] Jean-Paul Gaudillière and Ilana Löwy (2001: 3) argue that studies of statistical patterns of transmission using Mendelian inheritance became a focal point in the early 1900s, giving new shape to diseases such as hemophilia and Huntington's chorea. Through the concept of predisposition, many common diseases were placed in the purview of research on heredity.

This trajectory made asthma a potentially Mendelian disease in the twentieth century, and heredity became a subject of direct research. In 1913, two researchers based at a medical school in New York published a study on inheritance of allergic diseases, including asthma (Cooke and Vander Veer 1913). The purpose of the study, according to the authors, was to "determine definitely what part inheritance plays" in several allergic conditions (205). Family histories and clinical signs were used to determine this role of heredity. The results reveal the ambiguities of inheritance at the time: in the absence of precise concepts of transmission, the authors referred to what was inherited as a "tendency" toward allergies, an "unusual capacity for developing" sensitivity to foreign proteins (205). In cases where the condition skipped a generation, "It is apparent here that the parent not clinically affected has transmitted some characteristic to his offspring the nature of which cannot be specified" (211). However, this lack of specificity did not preclude the authors from stating that their results were sufficient "strongly to suggest that sensitization is inherited as a dominant characteristic" (218). This apparent discrepancy between the meanings given to what is inherited and the mode of inheritance reflects the use of Mendelian inheritance at the time, in which an unspecified locus was considered an active agent in shaping physical features (see Keller 1995; Kay 2000; Wailoo (1997: 143) notes a similar finding for sickle cell anemia in a study of families published in 1923).

In this disciplinary approach, inheritance became associated with a vague predisposition toward the allergic response that characterized asthma. Here, Salter's inheritance as particular to the neurosis type of asthma was inverted, and heredity applied exclusively to the physiological aspects of asthma. A 1916 treatise on asthma makes this transformation from Salter's view clear: "The individuals [with nervous asthma] exhibit from early infancy unmistakable signs of a functional disease of the central nervous system which is generally inherited, most frequently on the mother's side" (Berkart 1916: 16). The author goes on to delineate the sensory and motor nerve processes that are involved in the condition. Here, the gendered nervous disease of asthma is no longer a mental, emotional state as Salter found, but instead a purely physiological tendency.

This inherited tendency remained vague and capable of enigmatic effects. In 1930, a British physician wrote:

> In many cases the condition is familial in character, and inquiry will often reveal the fact that sufferers from the condition have been known in different generations. Thus heredity no doubt plays some part. Careful study in these cases will generally reveal some anatomical or physiological peculiarity which is more or less manifest in different members of the same stock. It may be a rickety tendency, or some dysfunction of the internal secretory glands, some tendency to particular metabolic disturbance, or some peculiar trait in the general "make-up." (Hall 1930: 9–10)

This transformation from asthmatic inheritance of an intrinsic neurosis to inheritance of some organic or physiological defect meant that the asthmatic with a family history needed physical treatment of the underlying cause of attacks, which in extreme cases included radical diets, prolonged exposure to X-rays, and cauterization of nerves. In other conceptualizations, this heredity was construed as a diathesis that must be present for asthma and other allergic conditions to occur. For example, according to a 1931 description of allergy, an inherited condition acts as a kind of potential, requiring emotional or other kinds of activation to become asthma: "Allergic responses may be precipitated by various psychological states but the allergic diathesis must be present first" (Bray 1931: 96). This interpretation of asthma as an allergic predisposition was attributed to Cooke and Vander Veer by subsequent researchers (e.g., Schwartz 1952), and formed the basis for the genetics of allergic disease.

Transformations in American and British medicine from the eighteenth and nineteenth centuries to the early twentieth century demonstrate the radically shifting meanings of concepts like heredity, blood, symptoms, and the causes of asthma. Histories that follow hereditary, or emotional, or physiological aspects of asthma as stable through different medical sources over the last three centuries mute this plurality. Such attempts to distinguish the actual from spurious characteristics of asthma identified by previous experts overlook the subtle shifts by which asthma has changed as an object of research and intervention. This history of contestation continues to be foundational to categories of asthma employed today. Heredity as a cause of neurosis became a physiological allergic predisposition. This inherited tendency also transformed from a cause explicitly of contrast—what was left over when no other cause could be located—to a nebulous force used to account for demographics. The role of blood in asthma etiology shifted from a part of lung respiration to a link between families that tend to have asthma. Treatments and definitions of asthma dialectically shaped each other, as asthma remained an uncertain and contested disease that linked emotions, diet, blood, and infection. Such integrated heterogeneity can be seen in medical approaches today.

Current Variations

Keirns (2004: 207) shows that after World War II, the allergists' view of asthma increasingly became the conventional one. In textbooks, asthma was a condition caused by allergic sensitization, with emotional conflict in the home addressed in some manner (179–80). In the early 1950s the oral steroid cortisone became a standard treatment for asthma. Keirns argues that, as with adrenaline, physiological response to the new medication was used as a diagnostic test, in this case distinguishing asthma from other lung diseases (209). In the 1960s, the disciplinary conflicts over defining asthma widened, as pulmonary researchers described lung tissue response and non-allergic asthma, and the concept of "infective asthma" became widespread (with consequent treatment by antibiotics) (208). In the 1960s and 1970s, new inhaled medications became part of the regimen, particularly the selective β2 agonists (what are today called "reliever" inhalers), and physiological response to this medication also became diagnostic.

This heterogeneity of techniques to categorize asthma persists in current medical texts and practices. Definitions based on atopy (allergic sensitivity) generally employ skin prick tests (testing the body's reaction to common allergens); measurement of total serum immunoglobin E (IgE) levels (amount of particular allergic antibodies in the blood); and/or measurement of the number of eosinophils (white blood cells involved in allergic response). Other research methods use questionnaires on patient histories of wheezing, cough, chest tightness, and breathlessness, often correlated with a physician's diagnosis. Some in the medical field criticize this technique as overly subjective: more objective alternatives proffered include measuring the response of the patient's lungs to the short-acting β2 agonist medication and to the allergen methacholine.[5] Severity is similarly divergently assessed, as self-reporting (Centers for Disease Control and Prevention 2002), medication use (Ungar et al. 2002), changes in peak airflow (Reddel et al. 1999), and frequency of emergency room use are all employed. The causes of asthma are similarly contested. Allergic sensitivity to pollens and emanations from house dust mites, cockroaches, and pets are considered an important part of asthma by most of the medical community. The role of airborne pollutants such as ozone is more controversial but also widely believed to be involved, particularly in asthma exacerbations. Cigarette smoke and other household behaviors including the use of cleaning products and perfumes are also thought to be risk factors. Food allergies, medical researchers have concluded, account for a very small percentage of asthmatics. The enigma of asthma results in considerable research and discussion comparing approaches to diagnosis, measurement of severity, and categorization (McConnell and Holgate et al. 2000; Tattersfield et al. 2002; Peat et al. 2001; Hunter et al. 2002).

The contested diagnosis and severity of asthma is accentuated by the private and public institutions involved in research and treatment. For the pharmaceutical industry, asthma ranks high in investment in research and education, owing to the large market for respiratory drugs. This interest results in research programs exploring genetic response to asthma medication (pharmacogenomics), economic advantages of different medications (pharmacoeconomics), and adherence levels to asthma regimens, in addition to the many educational programs and nongovernmental organizations supported by the industry. The high medical costs of poorly controlled asthma have led health care organizations to employ asthma management programs, in which pharmacy data are used to identify high-risk patients and doctor prescription habits are compared with recommended regimens. These industries also work with the National Heart, Lung, and Blood Institute (NHLBI), which funds several multisited studies on causes of asthma and a National Asthma Education and Prevention Program, which is designed to educate patients and health care professionals. Divergent meanings of asthma take shape through such research and intervention, in an admixture of public and private institutions and techniques.

These efforts have recently focused on the variability of asthma definitions as itself constitutive. The pharmaceutical industry and patient groups have employed the multiple concepts of asthma diagnosis and severity to argue for the inclusion of more than one technique, operationalizing heterogeneity. For example, studies have focused on the patient's experience of his or her disease to determine asthma diagnosis and severity: several such studies conclude that self-classification frequently underestimates severity, or that "mild" asthma is better considered "moderate" and "intermittent" is often actually "persistent" (Fuhlbrigge et al. 2002; Rand 2002). In other cases, the patient's perception is valued over other measurements in order to legitimize medical regimens: where one medication is less effective by one diagnostic criterion, it may be more effective according to the patient's view of symptoms. Low adherence rates for asthma medications are frequently cited as a significant cause for intervention in this context (Weinstein et al. n.d.; Apter et al. 1998; Bender 2002; Glauber and Fuhlbrigge 2002; Rand 2002): nonadherence is considered reason to expand the asthma management programs used by health care organizations; to market delivery technologies that are easier to use; and to increase prescription of medications with simpler dosing regimens. As a result, research on adherence rates explores patient beliefs and views about available medications, their dosage, efficacy, purpose, side effects, and mechanisms.

Pharmaceuticals have primarily replaced other treatment modes. The short-acting $\beta 2$ agonists are used for asthma attacks and are referred to as "reliever" medications. Inhaled steroids are used to prevent attacks and are prescribed for daily use (called "controller" or "preventer" medications). Oral steroids are used primarily in hospitals for acute attacks. Long-acting $\beta 2$ agonists are also used in connection with inhaled steroids for prevention. Other pharmaceuticals are available, including leukotriene receptor antagonists and older medications such as theophylline. Most recently, GlaxoSmithKline and AstraZeneca patented combination inhalers of the long-acting β2 agonists and inhaled steroids, which have become best-selling medications. These are reformulations of available medications, allowing extension of the company's right to exclusivity. GlaxoSmithKline's combination inhaler, sold as Advair in the United States and Seretide elsewhere, was the fourth best-selling drug in the world in 2004, according to the *New York Times* (Grady 2005). Immunotherapy (allergy shots) is still sporadically employed for asthma treatment. The market in pharmaceuticals and the different medications available have led to extensive research and interest in distinguishing medication response and expanding diagnostic criteria. The contested causes and accounts of the international increase in asthma discussed in the introduction reveal this continuing conflict over categorizing and measuring asthma prevalence, severity, and causes.

Asthma Genetics

The genetic approach to asthma occurs within the context of this disciplinary competition. Immunologists, pulmonologists, epidemiologists, and geneticists stake different claims to the space of asthma to be studied (e.g., in population demographics, lung response, immune systems, gene-environment interactions). The attempt to locate the genetic basis for asthma often involves reanalyzing existing studies; for example, genotype-phenotype studies are being conducted on data and subjects from the large-scale Childhood Asthma Management Program. Industry research is conducted primarily through collaborations between multinational pharmaceutical companies (e.g., GlaxoSmithKline, Merck) and biotechnology companies (e.g., Affymetrix). Some biotechnology companies, particularly DeCODE, are large enough to conduct such research independently.[6] As with other genomic research, asthma projects tend to involve academic and industry collaborations: for instance, the β2 adrenergic (AR) gene discussed earlier was discovered by a collaboration between the University of Cincinnati and Genaissance Pharmaceuticals. In 2002, a collaboration between a biotechnology company (Genome Therapeutics), a pharmaceutical company (Schering-Plough), and a research team at the University of Southampton announced results associating a gene (ADAM33) with asthma. Such research projects have resulted in several genes that geneticists argue influence asthma susceptibility, severity, and response to asthma medications.[7] Differing definitions of asthma are used in these studies, including IgE levels, response to β2 agonist, response to methacholine challenge, and physician diagnosis. These projects employ and thereby give shape to disputed meanings of environment-gene-asthma interaction.

The disciplinary disputes are attempts to settle the plurality of definitions of asthma found in American and British medicine over the last three centuries. This integrated heterogeneity makes stabilizing the category for study or intervention difficult, as patients, doctors, health books, researchers, and expert institutions offer competing perspectives. The contested causes, definitions, and treatments of asthma detailed above are diversely taken up in Barbados too, where some diagnostic methods (e.g., pharmaceutical response) are enhanced, and others (e.g., airflow measurement) are minimized, amid the biomedicalized focus of the state.

Chapter 4

(Re)Categorizing Asthma and
the Rational Pharmaceutical

Barbados has one of the highest levels of asthma of any country in the world, at 18–20 percent of the population, a number thought to be increasing sharply.[1] The following is a story about what these numbers mean. Asthma diagnosis, treatment, and prevalence estimates all vary widely as different criteria—some traditional, some more recent as a result of pharmaceutical and biomedical outreach—are employed in an expanding diagnostic approach to the condition. Biomedical and pharmaceutical practices discussed in the previous chapter are used in unexpected ways, creating new medical categories and techniques.

Detection and Intervention

According to a Barbadian researcher at the University of the West Indies, Barbados has a 19.8 percent prevalence of asthma, a seventeen-fold increase from 1973. The International Study of Asthma and Allergies in Childhood (ISAAC) found a 30 percent prevalence among Barbadian children in 1996, according to Barbadian asthma specialist Malcolm Howitt (cited in Greaves and Jarrett n.d.). Today, asthma is a primary focus of public health intervention, one of the five conditions for which Formulary medications are free, a source of media attention, and the object of considerable government outreach in partnership with the pharmaceutical industry. Patients diagnosed with asthma are prioritized at the polyclinic and the Queen Elizabeth Hospital (QEH) emergency room: as one polyclinic doctor, Emily Wraight, put it, "Complaints of asthmatics get right through because they are seen on an emergency basis at the polyclinics. So if they're asthmatic, they automatically go to the top of my list."

The classification of asthma is a recent development in Barbados. In the 1970s, bronchitis, or asthmatic bronchitis, or wheeze were the gamut of diagnoses for lung problems related to allergic reaction. Medical practitioners I interviewed described the change to early diagnosis of "asthma." Jeremy Rowe is the head physician of a polyclinic who focuses on asthma intervention. During an interview in his office, he talked about the shifting diagnostic techniques:

> There was a change in the way we defined asthma. Up until three years ago, we would make a diagnosis of wheeze, but it did not necessarily mean asthma. We'd call it "reactive airway disease." Before, a child who came in wheezing would be diagnosed with a chest infection. He would still be given medicine, but not diagnosed with asthma unless he came in again.

The shift to a more inclusive diagnosis emerged from the heightened attention by the government and pharmaceutical industry.

The National Drug Formulary is the state tool used to act on what is perceived as the asthma crisis. Of the medications for treating asthma available on the Formulary, the most commonly used are the following: inhaled corticosteroids and oral corticosteroids (both designed to prevent attacks); short-acting β2 agonists (designed for immediate relief from an attack); and the new combination inhalers. The government's public health approach to the condition is improved adherence to prescriptions and increased knowledge about medications. In this context, information about categorizing and diagnosing the condition comes from the interaction of the Ministry of Health (MOH) and pharmaceutical company outreach. "Asthma" has become increasingly inclusive amid this market and government pressure.

This recategorization of asthma complicates portrayals of a radically increasing rate in Barbados. Several doctors talked with me about patients being less afraid of the diagnosis, resulting in doctors being more willing to diagnose. Many talked about the new levels of awareness and information, both among medical practitioners and the public. Owing to this new focus, the increase in asthma is a highly disputed topic among health care practitioners in Barbados. Emily, who has a particular interest in asthma and diabetes, remarked, "We are *detecting* more asthmatics. It's hard to tell whether that's because there are more asthmatics or people are more aware. But we do see more, both adult and children." For these practitioners, asthma statistics in Barbados are opened to questions as patients newly identify with the disease and doctors change diagnostic techniques.

A variety of asthma diagnostic techniques are employed in Barbados, reflecting older methods (e.g., wheeze) and more recent pharmaceutical company emphases (e.g., medication response). Many physicians discussed the variation in diagnostic techniques across different medical facilities. At the polyclinics, wheeze alone was most often taken as a sufficient diagnostic. Private doctors employed a wide range of techniques, including wheeze, family history, and response to medication. Some practitioners criticized others who made diagnoses of a "whiff of asthma." William Anderson is a physician involved in designing health policy. As he told me during an interview, "Parents will come to you and say they know why they wheeze. The doctor told them it was a bad cold, or that they had a 'touch of asthma.'" William hinted at the antagonism that exists between different medical care sites: the perceived technological emphasis at QEH is contrasted with the traditional approach of private practitioners outside the public system. The polyclinic doctors talked especially about the lack of time, personnel, and technology for more elaborate diagnostics. Emily linked this problem to diagnostic contingency: "The polyclinics don't have the technology to make an objective decision. The protocols are not always followed. At the QEH they have technology, they can test objectively. In the polyclinics any who wheeze are treated as asthmatics. We don't have spirometers in the polyclinics, only peak flow meters." For many practitioners in the rural areas, this variation is not viewed as a lack; instead, the peak airflow meters that Emily implied as minimal were themselves considered excessive. A rural private general practitioner explained this position: "The techniques vary from place to place....I have a peak flow meter but I don't tend to use it too often. If I see a patient [he acts out wheezing], I don't have time to say, 'What's your peak flow and how much has it improved over a period?'" This doctor relied on the response to medication for diagnosis. Such variation in diagnostic techniques reflects economic and medical differentials between rural and urban areas. In the context of the increased attention on finding asthma, these multiple techniques allow for an expanding medical category.

Excess Diagnostics

The intense focus of the MOH and pharmaceutical industry on identifying and intervening on patients with asthma has created a hyperinclusive diagnostics. As Emily commented, "The polyclinics don't have spirometers. Patients presenting with wheezing are assumed to be asthmatic. Wheezing and asthmatic are thought of as synonymous, without doing a proper investigation." Response to medication is similarly used expansively. Measuring the response to a β2 agonist is a common biomedical diagnostic technique for asthma, as noted in chapter 3. However, such techniques change in medical practice, taking on new significance in disease categorization. The most frequent use of this technique in Barbados is to prescribe a reliever (β2 agonist) medication and if the patient describes getting better, then he or she has asthma. I talked with several private doctors who considered improvement with a course of β2 agonist medication to be diagnostic, as did this general practitioner, Donald Carlin: "I use history, and if they're wheezing, and—how you really know is with a therapeutic trial. If you do a therapeutic trial and the patient responds and the symptoms get better, that's your diagnosis. At the QEH or something they might use bronchial challenge or something like that but a therapeutic trial will tell." In an exchange with a pediatrician who used a similar method, I expressed my surprise at the incidence of asthma he had found:

NEIL: What incidence are people telling you?
AUTHOR: I mostly hear around 18 to 20 percent.
NEIL: [Nodding his head] I would say significantly higher. I would speculate 80 percent.
AUTHOR: Eighty?!
NEIL: [Nods his head again] Eighty to eighty-five. Of course it depends on how you define it. Asthma is a spectrum. I prescribe a drug not FDA approved that's made in Canada, called Berotec. It has a longer duration of action. Any child that walks into my office with a cough responds to bronchodilators. Ninety percent of kids who come in have asthma. Now, whether they develop a wheeze is another question.

This was by far the highest number I heard for asthma prevalence in Barbados, but the diagnostic technique of assessing response to pharmaceuticals usually led to exceedingly high estimates of asthma prevalence. Such biomedical techniques get used in ways not limited by their rationality, as market, traditional, and personal proclivities extend one another. The excess diagnoses emerge from the use of multiple traditional (e.g., wheeze) and biomedical (e.g., response to β2 agonist) techniques, combined with a pressure to locate and intervene on asthma.

The various criteria are each considered independently sufficient for diagnosis in an exaggerated diagnostics. The private general practitioner Thomas Lancaster, who practices in Bridgetown, employed such an inclusive set of techniques: "I diagnose on symptoms alone, nocturnal asthma responds well to asthma medications. I use wheezing. With older patients, I use the peak flow meter, a change in peak flow rate at different times. And in response to Ventolin [a β2 agonist manufactured by GlaxoSmith-Kline] so there are a variety of methods." An expansive category of asthma is thereby created. Elliot Woodward is the head physician of a polyclinic in a relatively urban area. He talked with me about the shift in diagnosis and his own methods:

> Diagnosis has changed over the years. There was a fear of being diagnosed with having asthma. We used to diagnose wheezing bronchitis, or asthma bronchitis, because these are more acceptable to people....For example, if someone comes to me with a respiratory illness—some people—my brother wheezes, my wife wheezes, I treat them as asthmatic even though they're not asthmatic. Even though they never wheezed before and don't wheeze regularly. I diagnose them as bronchitis with wheeze. And I prescribe for asthma. There's not very much in the literature about that.

This emphasis places pharmaceuticals in the center of not only asthma care but also the conditions, doing away with even medical diagnoses.

The Potential Asthmatic

This expansive approach is an object of considerable criticism in Barbados. In December of 2003, I attended a meeting about asthma. The meeting was designed to educate medical practitioners as part of a public health program by the MOH. It took place at one of Barbados's nine polyclinics and was attended by clinic nurses, environmental health officials, and physicians. After the physician who was head of the polyclinic spoke briefly about the increase in asthma in Barbados, another doctor spoke about the definition of asthma, common triggers, and pharmaceutical treatments. A level of frustration and impatience from the audience could be felt. When the floor was opened to questions, I was surprised at the number of hands that went up. The questions focused on determining who was actually asthmatic. After the first few questions, the hand raising was dispensed with, as members of the audience rapidly and loudly posed questions; after each question, others in the audience usually expressed their support for the question and an additional one:

QUESTION: Is it true some people are born with it, and grow out of it?
RESPONSE FROM SPEAKER: Once you are asthmatic, you are always asthmatic. Even if you have symptoms only once or twice, you are still asthmatic for life.

This answer provoked many critical responses among the crowd. Several said that this did not make sense; some continued to press the question: Can you not have it then get an attack later? This frustration came from a sense that the diagnostics were unclear, that amid the increasing education and outreach, it remained unknown exactly who the patient was.

Nurses were particularly suspicious of the dramatic increase in rates of diagnosis. In one interview, I talked about asthma with a group of seven nurses from a polyclinic in a northern rural area. As we discussed this increase, the nurses focused on the changes in labeling. They told me about the number of parents bringing in children who have been diagnosed asthmatic. One commented (to the assent of others), "Sometimes, a child is diagnosed with asthma, the reason he is coming by, the child is listed as asthmatic, but the child has never had an attack!" Several families and asthmatics that I met told me similar stories of being diagnosed with asthma prior to any attack; some never have had one. This creation of a "potential asthmatic" was usually based on family history.

Increasingly, heredity and genes are linked in diagnosing asthma, largely as a result of the attention given to the asthma genetics study. Kimberly Jameson is in her mid-thirties and a mother of two asthmatics. During one interview, we sat at a table in her home while her three young children played. She described the first time her son was diagnosed with asthma:

He had a bad cold, and then he started like coughing and he keep up constant crying and I feel that breathing was, like, uncomfortable. So I thought it was just a cold so I decided to take him to the doctor. And then after the examination, they told me that he was asthmatic. So they asked me if I have anybody in the family. So I told them his sister is, so they told me that it may be the genes are so close.

Recent medical practice in Barbados has seen a reframing of the family impact on asthma as "genetic," a concept without precise meaning for most practitioners. Genes in this discourse operate as vague objects that carry the disease from one family member to another.

This genealogical diagnostic at times results in the phenomenon of the potential asthmatic, as this young woman explained to me:

> I remember the first time I went to the hospital! But the thing is, I was diagnosed with asthma before I actually had an attack. I would have a lot of bad colds. The minute she [her sister] got a cold, I had a cold. So they were really persistent, especially with the coughing. So my mother had taken me to the doctor, and he had diagnosed me with asthma before the first attack. So when the first attack came, it wasn't a big surprise. It was something looming.

I heard several such stories of being diagnosed without having had an attack from other individuals, within and outside of the study. Asthma as "something looming" creates patient identities in the absence of any symptoms. One pharmacist I interviewed criticized the overreliance on heredity for diagnosing asthma, arguing that the category of the potential asthmatic results in diagnostic confusion and consequent nonadherence: as patients believe they are asthmatic based only on family history, they refuse to believe they are asthmatic unless a family member is diagnosed.

For many in the medical care system, asthma diagnostics in Barbados exhibit a kind of runaway biomedical emphasis. Approximately half of the physicians I talked with felt that the expansive diagnostic created overdiagnosis that accounted for the increase in asthma. The use of several criteria as independently sufficient particularly troubled this pharmacist: "A few years ago, my three children were diagnosed as asthmatics. But only one seriously showed signs—but only one really had it. I will see patients who have a little cough, and doctors will say it's 'a little asthma.'"

Aside from families of asthmatics I spoke with, the pharmacists were the most outspoken in their skepticism of the diagnosis of asthma. Many wanted more objective techniques, as Mitchell Baines remarked: "I would like to be aware of the criteria for diagnosis of an asthmatic at Asthma Bay." Often pharmacists and families explicitly link this overdiagnosis to pharmaceuticals. Leonard Adams runs a pharmacy in Bridgetown and is a father of an asthmatic. He told me, "The doctors here don't do proper diagnostics. They do what I call the 'Aah Baah' test. Say 'Aah,' say 'Baah,' write the prescription."

Ryan Pinch, who runs a large urban pharmacy, similarly tied prescriptions to an excess of cases. During an interview about practitioner diagnostic habits, he told me: "What they do is shoot wide, almost like antibiotic

treatment. If you have an allergy, there's a whole set of inhalers [and] neb-
ulizing is prescribed. If you come in with any cough or wheeze, you got
asthma. Everyone is got asthma." These criticisms of marketized medicine
(by individuals who sell medicines) cast doubt on the automatic route from
diagnosis to pharmaceutical consumption. As I discuss in chapter 6, families of asthmatics offer the strongest critique of this link.

The expanding diagnosis has been accompanied by expanding pharmaceutical intervention. One participant, describing the treatments she has
received for her asthma, gave an account involving seven doctors she had
seen, each of which tinkered with her regimen until she was simultaneously being prescribed seven different oral medications and three inhalers.
While this experience was exceptional, I routinely heard similar stories of
patients being switched to different medications by different doctors, often
involving returns to a previously discontinued medication. The ubiquity of
asthma pharmaceuticals reflects the focus of government intervention on
asthma. Such pharmaceuticalization is seen as intimately tied to the diagnosis of asthma, in a critique of biomedicine gone haywire.

Pharmaceutical Gifts and the State in Debt

At the asthma meeting I attended in which the diagnostic category was
critiqued, treatment was another controversial issue. The audience wanted
to know what to do about an asthma attack in the absence of an inhaler.
The speakers talked about the necessity of always carrying one's inhaler.
Several voices responded at once, relaying stories of patients not having
inhalers with them. One of the speakers replied, "Call an ambulance."
This provoked frustration, exasperation, and some derisive laughter from
the audience. One audience member remarked loudly, "By the time you
get to the hospital, you could be dead." Two other nurses followed with,
"You be dead by that time." I asked one sitting close to me, why? Three
turned to me to answer, two nodding as one explained: "The ambulance always break down, or it's always out." "Always," one joined in. The speaker's
focus on pharmaceuticals as sole intervention provoked frustration from
this crowd.

Asthma intervention in Barbados is largely shaped by multinational
pharmaceutical companies in an array of asthma education and health information at different sites. Literature about the condition is ubiquitous
in medical facilities. Pamphlets and posters produced by the industry are
found throughout private and public health care facilities. In almost every
general practitioner's and pediatrician's office I entered, and at the hospital,

advertisements for an asthma pharmaceutical were posted. The companies have annual meetings in which they launch new products; bring internationally recognized experts to lecture on conditions; conduct weekly presentations at the polyclinics; and conduct joint lectures and symposia with the MOH designed alternately for teachers, medical practitioners, and the public. In addition, they provide funding for nongovernmental organizations and MOH outreach programs.

In the perspective of many medical officials, a diagnostic category of asthma comes out of this industry involvement. As policy physician William Anderson told me, "Signs and symptoms here come out through public health with the private sector coming on hard and fast, because they're moving and want to get the medicines and literature out there." For William, medical diagnostics emerge from a hybrid of market and public medical knowledge, just as much as the Barbadian system of care described in chapter 2. Some state medical practitioners expressed their desire for further integration with the industry. Joan Dane, a polyclinic nurse involved in asthma outreach, discussed the importance of this involvement for health care. When I asked where the polyclinics get information about asthma, she talked about the support from pharmaceutical companies. I asked her what the companies did and she responded:

> Glaxo is very good. We get a lot of good materials from them. They do. But mostly they get involved if they have products to give to doctors. If there's supposed to be a big lecture, they will set up a booth, but we need it at the local level, to talk to patients. This year we had a trainer's program for doctors, nurses, and environmental health officers at each polyclinic. We're hoping to see asthma clinics in each polyclinic, and hopefully in the new year, we are getting one here. We had started that in the hospital, but it didn't work because they're going more to the polyclinic.

In Joan's view, shared by many doctors and nurses, the dearth of information was a gap in pharmaceutical company outreach to the patients—intervention at the local level is a health need to be filled by the market.

As noted, the companies pose such fulfillment as a charitable act. In interviews, pharmaceutical sales managers distinguished educational materials from detailing (the process of marketing products to physicians):

> With the [asthma product] we hold meetings throughout the polyclinics system and pharmacies for the mechanics of the [product]. We have small meetings with various doctors. We offer a portable spirometer for the doctor

to do asthma management. We either teach them how to do it, or we will go in and do it—we will come and interpret the scores and continue to support doctors, with CMEs [continuing medical education courses] and on. So we are involved in education that way.

This framing of education as a gift, in the sense Marcel Mauss (1990) gives us, is significant in both small ways (in making alliances with nurses and doctors in hospitals and private practice (see Oldani 2004)) and in terms of health policy, as noted in chapter 2.

The gift status of pharmaceutical company intervention comprises a rebuttal to accusations of market agendas. Elaine Graham, a pharmaceutical sales representative, remarked to me during an interview, "We are big on education, and other companies just want to sell medicines. I don't think [a competitor] has ever done the education that we do." For Elaine, the education programs are not only a gift to the public health system of the state but also an answer to the accusations of profane profit interests: she singles her company out as not simply looking for profits but instead offering a needed service. Another sales representative told me about her company's willingness to educate: "[Our company] is very ethically conscious." Within this logic, the education is dissociated from company interests. However, at times representatives link the education explicitly to marketing. Elaine described her approach to getting a new product into the market: "First you educate, then you shift to the new drugs." The charity of providing needed educational help to the state—an act posed as ignoring the market—facilitates the proper sale of medications, which is necessary to gain a competitive edge.

This gift of pharmaceutical literature is particularly salient for the polyclinics, where lack of funding and personnel is acute. As one general practitioner remarked to me, "Companies don't talk to the general public, but certainly for health care professionals they are diligent. The reps matter a lot." Pharmaceutical sales representatives were frequently considered to be providing a kind of public service. Hector Cole is head physician at a polyclinic in a particularly poor rural area. During an interview at his polyclinic, he talked about the need for this kind of work: "Companies offer a lot of patient information on asthma control and management. Especially at the polyclinic, where you don't have time, you hand them a booklet to say things you don't have time to say." In this pamphlet-as-intervention, the companies are again appreciated for filling a perceived gap in asthma health care. This gift exchange places the state in debt to the pharmaceutical industry.

Critiquing the Gift in Asthma Care

But, as I demonstrated in chapter 2, processes like pharmaceuticalization often do not proceed straightforwardly[2]: the recipients in Barbados
consider this gift tainted and dangerous. Health care workers repeatedly
stressed their misgivings about pharmaceutical company outreach as health
care intervention. Pharmacist Ryan remarked:

> Education is a serious problem when it comes to the chronic conditions, and
> education is when the drug companies are launching a drug. You will get
> seminars, pushing the drug, and very little information generally on chronic
> conditions. Except HIV. Very very little education on triggers, on preven-
> tion, of marginal or no significance. On the general populace, 90 percent of
> people don't understand prevention of asthma and there's very little in the
> public sector.

Ryan's sentiment toward the lack of discussion of prevention or practices
that set off asthma was echoed by many pharmacists and Barbadians not
involved in medicine. In another interview, he talked more about the role
of the pharmaceutical companies:

> I tend to wonder if their involvement is more to educate or to confuse. They
> tell you a lot about the arguable weaknesses of one drug over another. But in
> terms of the long-term effects of a drug? And the general public is not inter-
> ested or even able to understand these minor weaknesses. So the education
> has a competitive focus.

Crucially, however, this criticism does not preclude use of literatures from
the pharmaceutical industry. Ryan has two posters on the wall of his pharmacy for current asthma medications. Physicians also expressed such ambivalence. Polyclinic head physician Hector, quoted earlier talking about
using pamphlets as a form of care, hinted at some of the perceived ambiguities in this relationship. He continued, "How much does the average
person who does not know about their health get [from these pamphlets]?
Not much. There's not much health information per se." One influential
urban pharmacist remarked, "There's a lack of really good asthma education. It's not as patient-oriented as it needs to be, it's too much about product advertising." This simultaneous judgment and acceptance occurred
frequently, particularly among polyclinic and rural physicians. Pharmaceutical industry interventions were thereby implemented alongside critique
of their market interests.

Pharmacists and physicians skeptical of the influence of the pharmaceutical industry portrayed this unease as a necessary balance, similar to the way health care officials viewed it in chapter 2. In a discussion about this influence, polyclinic physician Jeremy Rowe remarked:

> Couple of issues. First, I have a certain amount of discomfort with their involvement. They're in business: they want a profit for shareholders, that's what they're about. We like to think we're—maybe not altruistic—but trying to help. It's a conflict of interest, providing information—[he points to a Pulmicort poster on his office wall] every time they see that, they see AstraZeneca, so next time they will ask for it. We try and find a place where our interests meet. And I try not to endorse any product or company, I don't go to their conferences, but the relationship is still one to be careful about. There are ways that they can help us.

As with the Formulary Committee members, the optimization of health was posed as only achievable through a vigilant yet cooperative relationship with the industry. He went on:

> Yes, drug reps are more involved. They listen more, they're more subtle now—a few years ago they were just interested in detailing the drugs and in this study. Now they spend more time, ask how you are, find out who you are, what issues you have, they'll say, "The last time I talked with you...." They give open offers, serious offers—"If you need information about the condition." They want us to perceive them as suppliers of information.

For Jeremy, the industry's provision of information is a strategic positioning. In another conversation, he talked about the utility of this process, because of the need for information in the polyclinics. The pharmaceutical pamphlets and detailing are almost the exclusive source of medical information, and are highly valued; yet this information is also distinguished from real health care information, in which other types of interventions would be included. But the lack of time and personnel, and the sophistication of the materials from the industry make such information a valued form of medical care.

Interestingly Jeremy went on to categorize this source of information with family and community as nonmedical sites of health discourse: "It used to be 'I will give you free samples.' Now, it's videos, teaching aides, whatever way they can find to sell their product. We like to think we are the main suppliers of information but we're dreaming. In any condition, including asthma, people get their information from friends, family members." Classifying pharmaceutical literature with family narratives framed both as inevitable to health care practices: the medical practitioner can only find ways to work around and with such extramedical interventions. Jeremy advocates a careful relationship with the pharmaceutical industry, perceived as dangerous in its efficacy, sophistication, and influence, but also one that can be mutually beneficial. Such are the ambivalent uses by which the pharmaceutical industry is incorporated into the particularities of medical care that define asthma and its intervention. Pharmaceuticalization of public health intervention occurs as moral and medical dearths are posited.

This uneven evaluation can result in unexpected reversals. Polyclinic physician Hector talked about private practitioners prescribing drugs not on the Formulary:

> The [private] doctors see these drugs, they think "great," but the average patient cannot afford to pay $50 a month. Some of the fancier inhalers, until they reach this book [gestures to Formulary]—A lot of private doctors see new medicines, and get excited. They don't know that the patients will come to us *after* coming to them. Patients are too ashamed to tell private doctors, "I can't afford it."

Hector's views reveal the broader tension between the rural and relatively less funded medical facilities and the more urban and well-funded QEH and private facilities. The rural practitioners pose their own techniques based on wheeze, or already available medications, as more valuable, more based in what Barbadian families want, as more in touch with their communities. These doctors place less emphasis on the newer medications (even those that are on the Formulary) and devalue new diagnostic techniques as unrealistic for widespread use in Barbados because of economic considerations, and as an excess of diagnostics. As a result, adherence is of less concern in these facilities, despite the fact that pharmaceutical pamphlets are more uncritically accepted as sources of medical information. The goal of multinational pharmaceutical companies is to increase the prescription of patented drugs. As Hector revealed, the spread of information from pharmaceutical companies can occur in opposition to such prescription. Thus, at the medical sites most conducive to pharmaceuticalization—where pharmaceutical company information is most valued and employed—the pharmaceutical company agendas with respect to inhaled steroids are least realized. Such are the ways processes like pharmaceuticalization occur ironically and unexpectedly, as multiple contrasting hierarchies are constitutive.

Alternative Readings

The asthma that takes shape in pharmaceutical literature incorporates medication response. The most common posters and pamphlets show a computerized image of the human lungs. The bronchial and airway tubes are depicted, and elsewhere on the forms are enlarged, with captions explaining the physiological effects of an asthma attack. This depiction was the most common reference point for discussing asthma among medical professionals I spoke with, with the exception of wheeze. This formulation places inhaled steroids into the meaning of asthma (depicting the physiological sites of their activity). I want to be careful to note here that I am not disputing this logic: I too consider inhaled steroids critical treatment for severe asthmatics. However, alternative ways of understanding asthma exist in Barbados and elsewhere, with different implications—for example, the spatialization of asthma as pollen distribution, or sites where dust mites and cockroaches are prevalent, or proximity to pollutants and hazardous chemicals. In the formulation conveyed by pharmaceutical pamphlets, the disease is a condition defined in terms of the physiological effects of the medication—that is, a lack is designed into the condition; the need for the pharmaceutical is already part of the meaning of the disease. This contrasts with other ways of understanding asthma in Barbados, reinforcing the instability of processes like pharmaceuticalization.

The areas requiring asthma intervention most commonly proffered by Bajan families as well as some physicians and state officials, were pollution and food. This view intrinsically differs with the pharmaceutical approach by including a search for the causes of asthma within Barbados, an issue about which families, practitioners, officials, and most others I talked with have strong opinions. The role of environmental factors in asthma is an object of considerable discussion, if not techniques or funding for studying or acting on them.

Since the 1960s, the country has shifted the basis for its economy from sugar to tourism, light manufacturing, and services (see Freeman 2000: 30). Since the 1990s, partially through economic policies of the IMF and the General Agreement on Tariffs and Trade (GATT) (and subsequently the World Trade Organization), tourism and foreign investment in particular have shaped economic policy (International Monetary Fund 2003 and 2004). The result has been a dramatic increase in automobile use, large-scale construction, and food importation. During my research among families of asthmatics, I was often told that there were more asthmatics in Barbados because of the "pollution," a term covering exhaust from vehicles, chemicals used as pesticides, and particles produced by roadwork. (In chapter 6 I explore the significance of these critiques of perceived modernization among the Barbadian families of asthmatics.) This discourse by the families and some health care workers led me to interview members of the government involved in regulating and monitoring these practices, including representatives of the Environmental Engineering Department and the Pesticide Control Board and environmental health officials. In these interviews, a state perspective on asthma emerged that differed from that discussed by members of the MOH. This is perhaps unsurprising: in the United States one hears different emphases on asthma at the NIH, the FDA, and the Environmental Protection Agency. The point here is that these discourses in Barbados are placed into conflict particularly as responses to the involvement of the pharmaceutical industry. The influence of the multinational industry is denigrated as representative of the same global markets that are causing asthma in the underprivileged country.

Medical practitioners and environmental regulatory officials portrayed Barbados's rapid integration into the global economy as creating a damaging excess of pollutants and pesticides. Polluted air, particularly from vehicle exhaust, is a ubiquitous topic of discussion around asthma in Barbados. As general practitioner Gregory West put it, "In Barbados the atmosphere is polluted, traffic has increased, I would say it's three times what it was five years ago." Raymond Pearson is a high-ranking official from the government agency that monitors motor vehicles. During an interview in his office, he talked with me about pollution and asthma:

Of course, Barbados is not as polluted as some other localities. But exhaust emissions has increased significantly. The number of vehicles on the road is now 90,000 to 100,000. This has increased significantly in the last 10 years, from 50,000 to 100,000, which means high exhaust emissions. Also, Barbados has an increasing amount of chemicals, aerosols, being put in the atmosphere as well.

According to Raymond, this results in increased diesel consumption and carbon monoxide levels in the air. He noted that his department has "decreasing activity on air pollution however, recognizing a higher population." As the government adapts to changes brought by global markets, such regulations become deemphasized. The traffic is also related to increased roadwork, which physicians in the urban areas discussed in particular as causing the rise in asthma. Raymond talked about asthma exacerbations caused by localized industrial activity such as quarrying and construction of buildings and roads. Dust is repeatedly talked about by families and medical practitioners in relation to asthma. Emily Wraight's polyclinic is next to a large road construction project, and she had documented the increase in the number of asthmatics coming to her polyclinic during periods of construction. As another doctor noted, when asked about demographics of asthma prevalence, "If we see clusters, it's because roadwork and construction is going on."

As officials and physicians reflected on this worrying rapid industrialization, they emphasized the poor as the group who experience the ill health effects. These people were more likely to be exposed to road construction and exhaust in the air. Raymond talked about the implications of increased traffic for individuals "walking the highways," referring to the generally poorer people who do not own automobiles continuing the tradition of walking along what are now heavy-traffic roads. Often these individuals are mothers carrying their children. Officials like Raymond, as well as many families, feel that this causes asthma in children.

These regulators and physicians discussed potential state interventions that they felt were underfunded or overlooked: reducing emissions, less reliance on diesel, reduction in the number of vehicles on the road, and better control of road construction—all lost in the focus on pharmaceuticals, in their view.

As integration into a global economy brings unclean air, it also brings unclean food, in the view of many Bajans. The economic changes have brought a rapid expansion of imported and processed foods, and a medical discourse implicates artificial dyes as a cause of asthma. As I discuss in chapter 6, this emphasis on diet and asthma is most robust and extensive among families, but a few doctors, pharmacists, and nurses shared it.[3] One pharmacist remarked, "Diet-wise, we are moving away from the home-cooked meal, toward fast food." A private general practitioner linked this trend to family economics: "There are a lot more processed and refined foods in their diet....Sweet potatoes, yams, are less utilized, because they are in fact more expensive. If there's a problem with money, which determines what you will buy, it's a lot easier to buy a lot of carbohydrates, a lot of additives." For this practitioner, lower economic status leads to generally weakened health through poor nutrition, including the increased consumption of processed foods.[4] Similar to the situation with air pollution, some pharmacists and most government employees in environmental sectors believe the effects of these changes in food and diet on asthma are insufficiently assessed. Paul Morgan is an environmental health official

I interviewed at a rural polyclinic. He saw the changing diet as strangely ignored by researchers:

> Our academics are arrogant. There has been a significant change in our diet over the last twenty years. We have moved from ground provision, from fruits, vegetables, what we call ground provisions, and backyard slaughter of chickens, to now Barbados has the highest per capita consumption of chicken of anyone else in the world. The diets have changed significantly. The average chicken factory will slaughter 18,000 birds per day, plus we import chicken....And now with the fast food, with a lot of dyes...

As officials talk of artificial preservatives and dyes, they also implicate increased consumption of other chemicals, particularly pesticides. Due to the prevalence of dengue, a considerable government prevention campaign has been launched that includes seasonal spraying of insecticides in neighborhoods. Families are told to leave the windows and doors open during these sprayings in order to allow the chemical into the house, and then to close the doors, to keep the insecticide in for maximum effect. Mosquito insecticides are also marketed for home use to prevent dengue. Raymond noted:

> The increase in chemicals is perhaps accompanying the standard of living that has improved, before we would use burning coils, now we see the use of, what I call, these sophisticated poisons, the mosquito sprays, and bug sprays....The Pesticide Control Board, which is an agency of the Ministry of Agriculture, regulates chemicals and is also supposed to regulate use. Use is not as tightly controlled as importation.

Raymond considered such pesticide use a possible cause of the increase in asthma. Environmental officials also noted the hazardous mixing of chemicals by families using cleaning products, as well as by businesses. Raymond talked about this practice growing as manufacturing and the use of new products have led to new chemicals being brought into the country and increased chemical waste, which he believed was polluting drinking water. A polyclinic nurse I talked with also discussed this problem: "We had a young woman who died of mixing cleaning chemicals. The chemicals, from doing housework all day, and *spraying*." Head polyclinic physician Jeremy Rowe summarized this consumption of chemicals and air pollutants and dust in his notion of a more "polluted society":

> There is a more polluted society here. There's more use of industrial cleaners, more construction, industries burning rubber, factories with exhaust. It

was investigated and there wasn't found to be a link, but the complaints kept coming and they didn't stop. There are pesticides in the home. Dengue is endemic, so now what a lot of parents do is spray then let the children back in.

Asthma in these accounts is a disease caused by "consuming modernity" in a sense: inhaling and eating the pollutants wrought by integration into a global economy. Medical talk of chemicals, dyes, and exhaust poses a site for intervention on these social and economic changes, that contrasts with the state's pharmaceutical focus.

But these environmental and pharmaceutical perspectives were not intrinsically mutually exclusive approaches. The public officials involved in enacting pharmaceuticals as interventions often shared these critiques and alternatives. Audrey Keyes, who talked about the need for social research, when asked what causes asthma in Barbados, remarked, "I think it's the foods, the dyes. When I was growing up, you didn't get all the corncurls. Now, even in the lunch pack, they get corncurls and the popcorn, and the sweet drinks." These officials, like public medical practitioners, implement the focus on pharmaceuticals for asthma intervention while noting the underexamined environmental causes and potential sites of intervention.

However, in the accounts of medical practitioners and officials involved in environmental regulation, pharmaceuticalization has undermined attention to asthma as a disease of modernization. They associate this dearth of interest in pollutants with the excessive focus on pharmaceuticals as public health intervention. Paul talked about why action around asthma in Barbados emphasizes pharmaceuticals and downplays preventive environmental measures: "The education is done by nurses, the majority of the persons in education are nurses, doctors, and if you're a hammer every box looks like a box of nails. If the nurse is doing it, they are all focused on the curative aspect." Medical practitioners and officials involved in environmental regulations reproved researchers for ignoring these causes. As one environmental health official remarked to me after talking about the harmful use of chemicals by businesses and families in Barbados, "No studies are being done on this!"

A similar criticism of the narrow lens of Barbadian medical care occurred at a seminar I attended about asthma education conducted for primary-school physical education teachers at the Pan American Health Organization (PAHO) headquarters. The PAHO building was the most lavish site for an asthma discussion of any I attended, excluding pharmaceutical company lectures. During the seminar, the facilitator asked the audience to comment on the meeting. One teacher talked about the increase in cars and pollution in Barbados. She continued, "Babies are being carried on the side of the road, and the cars and they're breathing all these fumes, and I'm kind of surprised no one brought up that point. That as a trigger. All I remember from the talk is Ventolin. It's imprinted on my mind." Asthma as a condition born of modernization represents a critique of that particular extension of modernization, pharmaceuticalization. The pollutants of modernization provide an often unspecified counterpoint to the restrictive positivity of the pharmaceutical-disease link posited by the industry. The perceived overemphasis on pharmaceuticals makes this a paradoxical modernity, in which the global commerce that creates the illness brings an obsessively narrow intervention on it.

But just as the agendas of pharmaceutical companies are at times reversed in their implementation, so pharmaceuticalization is not necessarily undermined by criticisms of the focus on drug efficacy. In the case of asthma pharmaceuticalization in Barbados, industry marketing utilizes such criticism. The industry posits the pharmaceutical as a social, economic therapeutic that acts on the problems of modernization identified by medical practitioners and officials.

Proper Consumption

The emphasis on pharmaceuticals in asthma intervention carries the consequent discourse on consumption of medication. Preventive health in this context means use of preventer inhalers (those that include an inhaled steroid). Adherence to a regimen involving inhalers is the central public health issue related to asthma in MOH lectures, education materials, and media accounts. A widespread underuse of these medications is proposed, and outreach to doctors and patients emphasizes increasing adherence. As a doctor at QEH explained to me, research conducted by the MOH has found that 60 percent of patients returning to the Accident and Emergency Department were nonadherent with their inhaled-steroid regimen. The attention on correcting this wayward consumption creates the specter of an irrational patient and a rational pharmaceutical.

In practitioner accounts, asthmatics stockpile oral steroids, refuse to take the newer and safer inhaled steroids, and overuse the $\beta 2$ agonists. Most medical practitioners and pharmaceutical company representatives argue that undue fear or beliefs are the cause of this inappropriate use of medicines. Veena and Ranendra Das (2006) draw on their work among medical practitioners and families in India to complicate such a discourse on compliance. They show that what are termed "irrational" compliance decisions involve pharmaceutical company and medical practices. As they note, the literature on adherence is often insufficiently attentive to systematic domestic economies, practitioner habits, and market irrationalites of prescription patterns (also see Trostle 1996; Kamat and Nichter 1998). Nancy Scheper-Hughes (1992), in her work on Brazil, similarly depicts a complex image of compliance that implicates international markets in family choices about medicine. Paul Farmer (2000) has drawn attention to the ways the problematic uses of medicines for tuberculosis and HIV are enmeshed in structural inequalities facing the poor: lack of access to education and ongoing treatment, gaps and problems in public health care interventions, and medical practitioner practices all contribute to this harmful consumption. I too present a story here that complicates the discourse on patient fears in adherence. Pharmaceutical companies, pharmacies, hospitals, and asthma outreach are involved in the variable consumption of medications in Barbados.

The figure of the asthmatic as a patient not taking the necessary medicine (or not being given the necessary medicine) constitutes a dearth of consumption. As polyclinic physician Hector Cole commented, "Some patients, rather than take the medicine, just show up at A and E [Accident and Emergency Department of QEH]. So they're at QEH with something that unfortunately could be resolved at home with inhaled steroids. And they don't go to the private doctor or polyclinic to get follow-up care. They wait till they get an attack." For these practitioners, nonuse of the medication is an irrational approach to medicine. As one doctor told me, "Patients take the drug emotionally." The inadequately consuming patient is the one who puts himself or herself in danger, or her child in danger. One physician compared not taking the medication to a fire in one's home. When I asked about how he achieved the adherence he had talked about, he told me, "I always tell people asthma is like a fire in the house. From the time you see you have a mattress on fire, you put it out, you don't wait until the curtains are on fire." The rational intervention of inhaled steroids in these accounts must (morally and medically) be imposed on an irrational sphere of desire, vagaries of household decisions, patient identities, and caregiver variation. The patients, the public, do what they want when they want, not what they should do if they were conducting proper risk analysis.

This dearth involves a moral responsibility as patient, as citizen, as mother. I talked with one nurse at the Asthma Bay of QEH while she helped patients with their nebulizers. She told me, "They aren't taking their inhaler. They get the steroid from the doctor's prescription. If they start wheezing, they come in. If their chest hurt, they just come here. They don't take on the responsibility of caring for themselves like they should. They've already been given the prescription. They come in when their chest hurts." This figure of an irresponsible patient is an object of rebuke, as was visible during an exchange I watched in the Asthma Bay. A patient came in complaining of wheezing. After talking to the patient about her condition, a nurse asked in a sharp tone, "And you only started taking the inhaler when?" The patient responded, "Three or four months." The nurse replied, with annoyance, "So for nine months you've had the trouble and you haven't taken an inhaler." Here, a studied asceticism was morally prescribed. The excess of patient use of state facilities like QEH was juxtaposed against the responsibility of proper consumption, in which a disciplined practice toward medicines is required.[5] Elsewhere, the responsibility was posed in terms of caring for children. In order to parent well, proper recognition of the dearth of medicine consumption was necessary.

In Barbados, this responsibility is linked to motherhood (I explore the use of this social role more fully in chapter 7). In the gendered domestic and medical economy, responsibility is unambiguously placed with the mother; this message was reinforced in pharmaceutical marketing pamphlets, in statements and practices around care by general practitioners and specialists, and among nurses and pharmacists. This process results in the mother of asthmatics as medicine facilitator, ambulance substitute, constant monitor, and director of preventive measures (e.g., diet restrictions, maintaining a "dust-free" environment, and minimizing contact with debris from roadwork and pollens). Doctors and nurses frequently countered the anger and requests from mothers they met in the emergency department with strong remonstrance about not using the medication correctly.

In the figure of the nonadherent asthmatic, rationality here has something of the meaning given to it by Max Weber, a cost-benefit, calculating, economic rationality of the ascetic worker. Medication consumption is discussed in terms of a labor force: experts estimate the cost of asthma to the Barbadian economy; the loss of workdays and bodily health is posed as a state burden. In government rhetorics and public research, the patient is an individual considered politically and morally responsible to consume medications appropriately in order to alleviate the financial burdens of the state: a kind of pharmaceutical citizen.

Side-Effect Silence

The irrational parent is particularly visible in discourses (and silences) on side effects. As discussed earlier in this chapter and in chapter 2, practitioners view pharmaceutical education as providing a kind of care, even though its contents are understood to be a troubled mix of information and marketing. In this context, explaining the side effects, efficacy, safety, and uses of the inhaled steroid is not considered the route to adherence because these are considered part of pharmaceutical marketing. Patient irrationality is considered intimately tied to fear. One private general practitioner told me during an interview, "There is a steroid phobia: [Parents think,] 'We don't want our children on steroids, steroids are bad.'" This view was widespread among general practitioners, pediatricians, and pharmaceutical representatives. Another private practitioner told me, "They don't like to accept the diagnosis. A lot of patients are in denial, they hope it is not asthma, they don't want the label. A lot are embarrassed, they don't like to walk around with the medicine. And they're also afraid of the side effects, there's a fear of steroids." A pharmacist mentioned an example of these fears: "Patients say, 'I don't want to take something that will weaken my heart.' There are urban legends that someone died with their inhaler in their hands." Another remarked, "There's a lack of knowledge by the older folk....Some people tell them if they use too much [inhaled] steroids they will get brittle bones."

The side effects of inhaled steroids comprise a disputed issue in international medical research. I cite here those listed in a GlaxoSmithKline insert for its combination inhaler: "Seretide Accuhaler/Diskus: Systemic effects may occur with any inhaled corticosteroid....Possible systemic effects include adrenal suppression, growth retardation in children and adolescents, decrease in bone mineral density, cataract and glaucoma." This information contrasts with that in a pamphlet written by GlaxoSmithKline for education in the Caribbean, entitled "Asthma? Questions and Answers":

> Inhaled corticosteroids are...similar to cortisol that is produced by your own body. The production of cortisol is your body's way of dealing with inflammation, stress, injury, and infection. Inhaled corticosteroids help the body's natural defense mechanism to reduce airway inflammation. Side effects for most patients taking inhaled corticosteroids are generally mild and may include thrush or hoarseness. The NIH asthma guidelines recommend inhaled corticosteroids as the most effective controller for persistent asthma.

This considerably different presentation was the one most likely to be read by general practitioners, pharmacists, and patients in Barbados. GlaxoSmithKline has an interesting dilemma of being motivated to present this positive view of inhaled steroids while attempting to differentiate the inhaled from the oral corticosteroid: oral corticosteroids are not produced by

GlaxoSmithKline and are commonly used by patients, competing with use of the inhaled steroids. The same informational pamphlet talks about the side effects of these competitors:

> Oral Corticosteroids are...given to you temporarily by an ER physician or your doctor to treat and reduce the most severe acute symptoms of asthma. Potential side effects of this type of steroid, when given at high doses for prolonged periods, include swelling, weight gain, brittle bones, and cataracts. The NIH guidelines on treating asthma recommend that your physician reduce or completely remove oral steroids from your treatment plan as soon as clinically possible.

These side effects are quite similar to those listed in the insert for the inhaled steroids. Medical practitioners and pharmacists rely on these company literatures in creating an image of a compulsively frightened patient-consumer.

Doctors take up the pharmaceutical industry approach to side effects, by avoiding discussion of them. One private family practitioner who treats relatively poor patients explained:

> I prescribe inhalers or systemic steroids. If a patient is having an attack, I go straight to systemic steroids....I prefer the Pulmicort Turbuhaler [a corticosteroid inhaler] because of the method of delivery....I tell patients, "Asthma will kill you, inhaled steroids won't." I explain, yes there are side effects, but I make a choice. I do give them some rationale.

This rationale was considered necessary given the temperamental parent as patient. In the conversation I had with the seven polyclinic nurses, one remarked, "Bajans only take medicine when they're feeling very ill. They are not medically oriented." Some classified this lack of medical orientation as "cultural," as did this pharmacist: "And there's fear of steroids, both oral and inhaled, for the younger people. With the older asthmatics, compliance is better, but they experiment with other things. Again, it has to do with cultural background. What is culturally acceptable. People who are not doctors tell them to use bush leaves." This cultural life is posed against the logic of preventive medications.

Adherence was dissociated from pharmaceutical company practices through this positioning. As discussed, the physicians and pharmacists had a strong critique of the pharmaceutical industry's influence on health care. But this judgment of undue powerful interests imposed on a public system was not linked to lack of adherence and patient practices; these latter are made cultural and gendered, caused by inappropriate fears.

The Rational Pharmaceutical

In the most recent twist, the pharmaceutical is represented as an intervention on these social, economic, and personal vagaries of consumption. Owing to expired patents, multinational pharmaceutical companies are attempting to shift such preventer inhaler use from inhaled steroids and long-acting β2 agonists used separately to the combination inhalers. As Ulrich Beck (1992) argues, risks are market opportunities. In the absence of unequivocal evidence showing better efficacy or safety than the available medications, GlaxoSmithKline and AstraZeneca position the combination inhalers as improving adherence. This rhetoric is increasing in medical literature as the pharmaceutical industry turns to marketing new formulations of already available drugs. As the fourth best-selling drug in the world, this positioning of GlaxoSmithKline's Seretide (and similarly, AstraZeneca's Symbicort) is critical to medical use.

Symbicort made it onto the Formulary in 2003, as did Seretide in a more provisional way. Symbicort was very quickly picked up by urban-area private and public medical practitioners in particular. As one public-system pediatrician told me, "All the children over ten I put on a combination inhaler." This speed of integration reflects the ways the pharmaceutical companies are the source of not only medication information but also expertise. In order to launch their products, GlaxoSmithKline and AstraZeneca conducted (competing) conferences meant for specialists and general practitioners, which I attended. Such conferences, bringing in international experts, are highly influential in Barbados, sites where family doctors and specialists learn about conditions and medications. These meetings are also part of the way pharmaceuticals are brought onto the Formulary, as Bajan doctors become advocates for their inclusion.

Both of these meetings were exclusive events and well attended. From discussions I had with audience members, it was clear that a level of prestige was associated with the invitation. The lectures occupy that amalgamated space of education and marketing, in the medical practitioners' view. Attendees commented on the product goals of the lectures but also considered these forums a primary source of information and lauded the status of the lecturers and sophistication of the materials.

The combination inhaler in the industry presentation was a rational intervention on nonadherence. Part of the rationality is to reduce the complexity of medical care: the pharmaceutical insert given to us at our tables at one conference described the product as "simple and convenient asthma control for your pediatric and adult patient." The speaker talked about "how to make asthma treatment simple." During his lecture, he explained the elevating stages of complexity of asthma intervention: "First we administer the correct medication. Then we make sure they are taking the medication. Then we go into the home to do environmental changes. Because this is complicated. The first is simpler, the second is expensive." This speaker explicitly suggested the relevance to Barbados as a poor country: in his view, given these economics of medical care, going into the patient's home is not viable. He went on: "We are trying to be simple: talk to the patient about what is achievable, what is acceptable. You cannot say, 'You must move.' It's easier for patients to use one device." The pharmaceutical was here a kind of social medicine, reducing the complexity of structural interventions, cheaper than moving families, or implementing pollution changes, or going into the patient's home. The combination inhaler is the vaguely economical-through-simplicity response for poorer countries.

At the second meeting, there was a similar emphasis on simplicity as the defining feature of the product. The presentation also focused on "empowering the patient," a common discourse in pharmaceutical advertising and medical outreach today, with adherence as the vehicle of self-empowerment. Such logic allows the irrationality of the patient to become an asset, by producing a medication that accommodates the variation and vagaries of (individualized)[6] patient desires.

The new product is presented as a tailoring of the medicine to the patient's wants, to those parts of the patient's life not found in the rationality of clinical trial endpoints. One piece of literature given to us at the tables during the conference elaborated:

> Although such an approach may seem less objective, and therefore less reliable than clinical measures such as lung function, this information does give GPs a clear idea of how patients perceive their own asthma....Asking patients relevant, simple questions such as whether their asthma affects daily activities such as sport, walking or housework, may reveal more about its effects on quality of life than relying on tradition medical end-points such as lung function and use of inhalers.

A product that responds to what the patients say they want in contrast to the "traditional" reliance on simple clinical tests incorporates social critiques of biomedicine: American and European social movements valuing patient experience in opposition to a depersonalized and hierarchical medicine are here integrated to make such experience an asset of the product.

The medicine that increases compliance becomes an intervention on a whole new set of social, economic, political, medical dilemmas: the pharmaceutical now acts on the variables of medical consumption—for example, socioeconomic status, medical practices, and patient identities. Making the product an intervention on consumption, comparable to an intervention on physiological outcomes, allows for new kinds of studies in support of product use. With this approach, pharmacoeconomics has become increasingly significant: studies of the ways pharmaceuticals save money for the health care industry, the national economy, or particular hospitals are used to support medications as interventions (for examples of such studies on combination inhalers, see O'Connor et al. 2002; Price and Briggs 2002). The combination inhaler is taken to intervene on problematic medical quandaries such as asthma management, doctor-patient relationships, and lack of health care infrastructure or personnel.[7] The pharmaceutical tightens the link between the person and the state. These medications are represented as responsive to cultural values, patient desires, lack of self-discipline: a social medicine pharmaceutical.

The Irrational State

As Michel Foucault demonstrated, institutions, individuals, and techniques are organized around discursive objects; in Barbados, the social medicine pharmaceutical is the product of the integration of multinational pharmaceutical industry interests, public health intervention on adherence, and media attention on patient consumption. And as Claude Lévi-Strauss conveyed, discursive objects are effected, indeed *are* only in systems of meaning: contrastive signs that are exaggerated or experienced in relation to other cultural categories, keeping competing meanings in play. Like the social medicine pharmaceutical, the pharmaceutical citizen is only possible amid its own undermining: it is deployed where gaps and problems in public health are acknowledged, a figure ubiquitous in medical expertise that is at times questioned, placed into quotes as indicative of a fervently market-oriented approach by the state.

Many physicians saw troubling medical care habits in medication consumption. Thomas Lancaster talked about prescription habits:

People access systems according to their experience. If a person comes in with a respiratory infection and I prescribe an antibiotic, I will generate a demand. The next time they have a cold, they will come for an antibiotic, un-less time is spent to teach them how to use their inhaler, how to manage their asthma, rather than just go to a doctor or polyclinic. I tell them regular use of inhaled steroids comes when you're well too.

Several doctors, in explaining why patients act "irrationally," echoed Tho-mas's suspicion of prescription patterns. Pharmacist Ryan posited a state with a kind of cultural orientation toward pharmaceuticals: "Ventolin and Becotide [an inhaled corticosteroid manufactured by GlaxoSmithKline] are widely used in the public system. They are part of the cultural language here." For many pharmacists and patient families, overemphasis by the state on consumption of patented pharmaceuticals is the reason why patients do not take medications as directed. As Ryan put it:

> It's overprescribed. Simply because it's free, doctors ubiquitously will write for it. So if the patient has an upper respiratory infection, they will get pre-scribed inhalers straightaway, when the primary problem is allergies. Because we had a few noted asthma-related deaths, doctors have become overly cau-tious. So they will prescribe all the inhalers, and nebulize for wheeze.

Ryan argued that in this excess of treatment, patients make their own deci-sions of when to use inhalers. Other families and pharmacists (as well as some nurses) saw this overprescription as the result of the excessive focus on unequivocally diagnosing asthma. In their perspective, the influence of the drug industry in Barbados resulted in the framing of an episode of wheezing as requiring harmful steroid consumption. Amid the posing of the pharmaceutical as a rational intervention, this counterdiscourse sug-gests an irrational state in which pharmaceuticals are used zealously.

The new combination inhalers are a particularly salient symbol of this compulsive medicine, for many. National Formulary Committee member Silas James talked about the decisions to make the combination inhalers free:

> I was against Symbicort going on Formulary. Because of the cost factor. We need to look at the cost-effectiveness. We are asking drug companies to sup-port our program. Symbicort is purely cosmetic. And I appreciate the com-pliance aspect, one inhaler instead of two. I have been an antagonist and have not been very popular for my position.

Silas here relied on an economic model to critique the influence of phar-maceutical interests on public health. For Leon Castor, a pharmacist and former drug sales representative, the combination inhaler symbolized the informal exchanges that emphasize an excess of patented drugs instead of proper medicine:

> I don't see why it should get on Formulary. It's lobbying. There are doctors who are consultants to Glaxo and they have influence with the Tenders Committee. And they're saying give them the strong, the Pulmicort [an inhaled corticosteroid]. So then a doctor will take a patient who's been on Becotide, and has no problems, and will say you need something stronger.

He later linked this process to patenting:

> Most brand drug companies are thinking about how to extend patents. The combined inhalers, they're extending patents because they're too skillful at marketing, so now on the combined inhalers you can't come down to the lowest dosage that is suggested for inhaled steroids.

Pharmacist Mitchell Baines echoed this view:

> There has been a continual increase in asthma medicines sold—more inhalers, more steroids. They're not making any new inhalers—instead, they combine the inhalers, which is not necessarily a good thing. They do it to protect their patents. Patients do not necessarily need to be treated with a steroid consistently. Sometimes they're alright on the reliever, but with the combination that's impossible.

These critiques invert the concept of the rational pharmaceutical acting on the irrational patient: here, an obsessive focus on patented drugs, produced by the informal exchange between the state and industry, creates a harmful use of medications that the patient must contend with. Such a counterdiscourse precludes an image of pharmaceutical company agendas as determinant: as competing medical discourses avoid such ossification.

Pharmaceuticalization and Genetics, Othered

I have explored here the strange phenomena produced by compulsive use of biomedical categories around asthma: side effects silence, potential asthmatics, 80 percent prevalence, social medicine pharmaceutical are all created out of this biomedical culture. And these phenomena have an effect. Treatment regimens, patient identities, government interventions are all organized around them. The multiple criticisms of and reflections on these processes by their practitioners reveal the instability within such systems. As the figure of the potential asthmatic proliferates, it is at the same time criticized by physicians as resulting in harmful use of inhaled steroids. As pharmaceutical literature is portrayed as necessary to fill gaps in medical care, it is simultaneously denigrated as market-driven. The result is moments of reversal and ambivalent processes of pharmaceuticalization. These twists and turns occur because critical reflections on categories and discourses are integral to their significance. Pharmaceuticalization is implemented by individuals who critique the process in which they are engaged.

This intricate relationship to multinational medicine is the context in which asthma genetics research occurs. The recategorization of wheeze into a biomedical definition of asthma happens in conjunction with the research. The genetics of asthma is incorporated into the expanding diagnostics, and race-disease links are given new salience. Evaluations of the genetic research by facilitators of the study and by medical practitioners echo the ambivalent views of the international biomedical interventions described in previous chapters. As the genetic research is taken up by the public health care system, figures like the potential asthmatic are given genetic and racial meanings, even as such research is criticized. As I will argue, the new diagnostics and evaluations produced by the research both suggest geneticization of race-disease links and reflect surprising alternatives to this process, as in the case of pharmaceuticalization discussed in this chapter.

Chapter 5

Biomedical Partnerships
Making Genetics Significant

The asthma genetics study is now one of several genetics projects in preparation or being conducted in Barbados by teams from Johns Hopkins University. The genetics of acute lung injury is being researched by a multisited U.S. collaborative effort that now involves a Barbadian researcher. A project on the genetics of obstructive sleep apnea is being conducted by a Johns Hopkins researcher and Barbadian doctors involved in the genetics-of-asthma study. Research on the genetics of dengue fever and on the genetics of asthma severity are extensions of the asthma study, involving several of the same facilitators. These studies involve exchanges between U.S.-based genetics researchers and Barbadian researchers/facilitators. As researchers and facilitators negotiate the relevance of this high-technology science to the postcolonial country, new medical approaches to race, genes, and care are created.

Medical Exchanges

In a conversation I had with a Barbadian researcher, he explained the reason why so much collaborative international research occurs in Barbados by citing an example: "The two met at a conference. One had access to the patients and the other had contacts with funders." Genetic research is premised on access to a population (i.e., the ability to get blood samples or other biological materials and some form of medical information by questionnaire or records). The existence of a stable and extensive infrastructure of nurses and physicians who can facilitate recruitment is critical to such research[1] (an often underemphasized bureaucracy). The attraction of the access to patients in Barbados is matched by the robust administration of the health care system. As one member of a research team explained about a particular genetics study, "We have to look at the pathology to get names, then contact the doctor to get permission. When the doctor gives permission, then we can contact the patient." These practices require networks of complete medical records and consistent contact.

The reciprocal value of the collaboration for the Bajan researcher is access to genotyping technologies, diagnostic machines, and funding. For example, at a meeting on the genetics-of-obstructive-sleep-apnea project, a Bajan researcher noted that the Queen Elizabeth Hospital (QEH) rejected his requests for a diagnostic laboratory to explore sleep apnea. The result of the meeting was that the Johns Hopkins team would explore providing the sleep lab and funding while the Bajan physician would facilitate purchase of the polysomnography equipment and location of the lab. This access to technology is not necessarily direct: often the U.S. researchers are valued as the mediators rather than the providers of diagnostic technologies, by conducting genotyping in the United States. For example, in the case of the dengue study, plans were made for genotyping to be done at Johns Hopkins for unrelated studies already in progress by the Barbadian researchers. The expertise and technological sophistication of the U.S. teams are accentuated in these agreements, for the Barbadian researchers. Prestige is critical here: as one of the leading biomedical facilities in the world, Johns Hopkins carries the significance of having the most current biomedical knowledge. In addition, the teams offer training of medical staff involved in the studies: by collaborating with the geneticists, doctors and nurses are often flown to the United States to receive training in study protocols, medical procedures, and use of technologies. For the acute lung injury study, plans were made to bring Barbadian nurses to Johns Hopkins for training in study facilitation and to bring internal medicine residents at QEH to Johns Hopkins Hospital to observe internal medicine practices there. This expertise is of particular value to Barbadian physician/researchers both to facilitate the study and to improve medical care.

The genetics team emphasizes the high technology, high speed, and large scale of genetic research in making the studies relevant to Barbados (on the significance of such a discourse to genomic funding and research, see

Fortun 1998). The acute lung injury (ALI) study is part of a Consortium to Evaluate Lung Edema Genetics, which includes the Medical College of Wisconsin, University of Tennessee, and Emory University in addition to Johns Hopkins. As the team noted, the collaboration is designed to create "the world's largest bank of DNA from patients with sepsis and ALI."

This image of vastness is supported by the expansion of research seen in Barbados. As discussed in chapter 1, the peculiar efficacy of genetics allows the integration of databases from studies of unrelated diseases, and a consequent ability to multiply research on a population to include different conditions. The Barbados studies overlap at several points. Most of the physicians and nurses are involved in two or more genetics projects, and the crossover in patient recruitment and study facilitation here drive the research. The genetic studies on sleep apnea and dengue recruit individuals from the asthma genetic study, through an additional questionnaire. The dengue research group found during preliminary investigation that a study on the genetics of dengue was already occurring in Barbados, conducted by a researcher from London. The projects thereby operate by a kind of involution that reinforces the impression of a rapidly expanding science that is the future of medicine.[2] For the Barbadian facilitators, this brings sophisticated technologies and knowledge into the troubled postcolonial state's medical system.

Populations and Care in Collaboration

The medical partnerships form through mutual attempts to represent opportunities. As the genetics team meets with private and public doctors, they accentuate the technologies that they bring and lists of genes associated with prevalent conditions(and deemphasize difficulties in making strong genetic associations, which they elsewhere explore, e.g., in team meetings). The Barbadian doctors in turn draw attention to the large number of potential patients and the administrative sophistication of their institutions, needed to facilitate such complex research. I attended a meeting at QEH between three Johns Hopkins researchers and a Barbadian physician, Taylor Newton, to discuss a potential study on the genetics of asthma severity. Taylor talked about the high prevalence of asthma, as indicated by visits to the hospital, mentioning the 10,000 asthma cases in 2003. He also discussed the history of asthma care in Barbados. He first focused on the problematic former treatment practices: "[At the Accident and Emergency Department] we would just make a circle of terbutaline and go to each patient, adrenaline, adrenaline, adrenaline, all around." Contrasting this practice with the current sophisticated strategies used in the Asthma Bay and modern medicines, Taylor emphasized the progress made by the hospital in asthma care, making his case for Barbados as the site of the genomic research. In the acute lung injury study, the Barbadian researcher indicated the utility of the hospital to the collaborative project by discussing the fact that sepsis accounts for 20 percent of the intensive care unit admissions annually. In these interactions, the Bajan practitioners frame the patient populations as potential international genetic participants and a sophisticated Barbadian health care system well positioned for such research.

But for the exchange to work, this emphasis on capability must be complemented with areas of need. In a delicate play of countermovements, Bajan practitioners present the care in Barbados as considerably better than that on other Caribbean islands, while simultaneously indicating the problems and deficiencies produced by lack of funding and technologies. This included the difficulties of there being multiple techniques of diagnosis. During a conversation about the dengue genetics study, Taylor remarked to the genetics team, "There are a lot of things that are called dengue here that are not dengue." At the meeting between Taylor and the geneticists studying asthma severity, Taylor emphasized the variation in asthma diagnosis among general practitioners, referring to the diagnosis of "bronchial asthma" or a "whiff of asthma." This led to a conversation about diagnosis in the Accident and Emergency Department:

> JOHNS HOPKINS RESEARCHER ERIC REID: Are there any competing diagnoses?...Who picks the label [whether it was] asthma or cough, who picks?
> TAYLOR: We will see them. We currently use the GINA [Global Initiative for Asthma] guidelines. There is a type of asthma, cough variant, I think exists but some of my colleagues don't.

I took Taylor's reference to the cough variant as a request for clarification from the researcher on asthma diagnosis. He here conveyed the hospital as the preeminent source of diagnoses in Barbados while noting areas where further expertise (such as the genetics team's) would help. At this point in their conversation, another Johns Hopkins researcher, Mary Warner, joined in by asserting the validity of the hospital diagnosis: "I have to say that what is called an asthmatic here who has then gone into our study has always been an asthmatic, which is a testimony to the diagnostics here." Exchanges such as this mutually stabilize particular techniques of asthma diagnosis and categorization: the hospital technique is both relied on and validated by the genetic research. Treatment regimens are also explored in these interactions. Taylor's (possible) request for expertise was later brought up more explicitly, as he asked about the role of antihistamines in asthma care, owing to some strong interest among his medical staff in this form of treatment.

Through this depiction, Barbados's attractions as a site for the genetic research are presented alongside the potential areas for Johns Hopkins to contribute. Eric asked Taylor about hospital records of visits to the Asthma Bay.

ERIC: Is it feasible to get an ER record review?
TAYLOR: Seven years ago we began a computerization process for A and E [Accident and Emergency] [but have never put it into place].
ERIC: At Hopkins we are looking at the data on labels on outpatients.

Eric suggested the possibility of Johns Hopkins creating a computerized system for the hospital to register outpatients. Collaboration with the researchers results in such new kinds of care and infrastructure for the Barbadian health care system. In the ensuing conversation, Taylor focused on this pragmatic utility of the biomedical studies: "You will percolate my interest when the genetics translates into medical care at my front door." Eric responded by referring to the registry system Johns Hopkins would provide. He then talked about recruiting patients for studies on asthma care: "I'm not talking about drug trials, I'm talking about tracking [emergency department visits] for follow-up care." As the Johns Hopkins researcher and Barbadian physician attempt to draw each other into the project, the U.S.-based genetic research is represented as not beholden to financial incentives while becoming a part of the Barbadian public health system. These exchanges create new medical diagnostics and infrastructures in Barbados.

But this flow of expertise is not unidirectional. The genetics team looks to the Barbadian researchers not only for patients and study facilitation but also for knowledge of the specificity of Barbados. The high levels of asthma and other conditions (hypertension, glaucoma, obstructive sleep apnea) cited by Barbadian researchers—comparable to those found among African Americans—are interpreted as linking the Barbados populations with those in Chicago, Baltimore, or other U.S. cities. One geneticist talked to me about the scientific opportunities of studying gene-environment interactions and asthma in Barbados, citing statistics on allergens brought by winds from Africa correlated with levels of asthma from a Barbadian researcher at the University of the West Indies. Through these interactions, as the meanings of disease and genetics and care are transformed for the Barbadian researchers, the meanings accorded to Barbadian patient populations and environment shift for the genetics team.

Genetic Futurism

Claude Lévi-Strauss (1969: 84) notes that in gift exchange, "the agreed transfer of a valuable from one individual to another makes these individuals into partners, and adds a new quality to the valuable transferred." The collaborations by which new biomedical technologies, expertise, and training are interpolated into Barbadian medical research generate new concepts of disease etiology, medical treatment, and who is a patient. The study facilitation meetings are one site of such negotiations between researchers and medical practitioners; conferences are another.

The Johns Hopkins–Barbados Genetic Epidemiology of Obstructive Lung Disease Research Conference took place in Barbados in 2004. This conference, conducted by the genetics teams, was designed to share the research and to recruit any medical practitioners interested in becoming involved in the studies. AstraZeneca partially funded the event and attendance was high, with an audience primarily composed of general practitioners and family doctors. The genetics teams gave four presentations (with extensive question-and-answer periods) on the genetic studies into acute lung injury, obstructive sleep apnea, asthma, and the environmental aspects of childhood asthma. The interactions between researchers and Barbadian medical practitioners at such meetings are highly influential, as I found in conversations with general practitioners and specialists discussing a range of diseases.

The lectures emphasized the scale and speed of genetic research. In the presentation on acute lung injury, the geneticist remarked, "What we are definitely advantaged by is that the Human Genome Project has led to these wonderful advances in technology: we can look at SNPs [single nucleotide polymorphisms] faster, we can do more gene expression, we can look at all of the genes at one time." These accolades link the Barbados collaborations to other international research by which the biomedical future is being created. He continued, "These technologies don't mean a thing unless you have clinicians to marry this technology to what's happening in the clinic." The concern expressed by Taylor about the lack of medical applicability of the genetic research is thereby addressed, as the medical practitioners become active participants in the utilization of new technologies. The conference presentation on asthma genetics also focused on the scope and speed of emerging technologies. Mary emphasized the complexity of asthma as involving multiple genes and gene-environment interactions, necessitating the candidate gene method adopted by the Barbados Asthma Genetics Study. She talked about the study finding an association with asthma in the chromosome region of 12q, noting, "STAT6, IFNG, MYPT1, BTG1...are examples of many, many candidate genes in this region."

This emphasis on the scale of discovery and the sophistication of technologies accentuates the potential of medical genetics: the research has uncovered various factors, analyzable through genetics, that affect the experience of disease populations such as Bajan asthmatics. The medical unknown of conditions like asthma becomes knowable through interpreting and utilizing the results of various genetic research projects. To use Bruno Latour's language (1999), the medical practitioners will better understand and intervene on the widespread presence of asthma among their patients by passing through the U.S. genetics laboratory. Mary discussed the team's use of higher-throughput genotyping technology produced within months of the presentation, allowing a scale of genotyping impossible in the past. As with the acute lung injury project, this mass of information is reinforced by the scale of the projects, as the data are made available electronically, "so that any investigator anywhere can conduct a blood test for a gene of their choice." The direction of this scale and scope of research is indicated by the sense of possibility: "We're just beginning."

The American researchers portray the research as international, fast-paced, and inevitable while simultaneously being responsive to the medical needs of a resource-poor postcolonial country. The Bajan facilitators present the areas of needed assistance to the high-funding and high-technology U.S. team, while portraying their own sophistication as an attractive site for medical research. This play of wants and offers is a postcolonial government's response to the discourse of genetics speed and fecundity. Medical practitioners in resource-poor countries like Barbados work to attract such research in order to gain from the promised medical future. They simultaneously portray their need for such expertise and their ability to contribute in a process of utilizing and adapting to this biomedical future. These reciprocal countermovements comprise a foundational mix of criticism and hope in the genetic future. As I learned, facilitation of the research does not necessitate enthusiasm for it.

Inevitable Genetics

The study facilitators and wider medical community of Barbados find the representation of genetics as the future of biomedical research convincing. The lectures, medical literature, and increasing number of studies being conducted in Barbados combine to make a strong case that medical genetics is a burgeoning international field that is increasingly shaping medical knowledge. In interviews, most general practitioners and pediatricians lauded this move and its potential impact on conditions such as asthma. I interviewed one general practitioner who has a private practice in an eastern rural area. She advocated further genetic research: "The role of genetics—we've come to the point where everyone believes it's part of the atopy, atopic reaction, but I would like to go beyond that and see what type of atopic individual would have asthma." Melinda Davis is a public health official I interviewed at her office at the MOH. She explained the utility of this research for intervention: "If you know a variety of things cause a problem, and if you can decrease one, then you have an impact. Genetic counseling—if genetics is one of the causes, and I know that, then I can take medicine, or I can know that if I marry someone who has asthma, 100 percent of our children will have problems." Such an account of a particular potential intervention based on the genetic research was extremely rare: doctors and nurses instead focused on the value of extending knowledge of a complicated disease.

But several doctors I interviewed had doubts. One general practitioner remarked, "Genetics is one of those areas that a lot of people are still skeptical, and rightly so. We need to get years of use first." A family doctor similarly found use in the clinic unlikely: "With genetics, I am waiting to see it put into practical use. A lot of people come and talk about asthma genetics here, and the study is being done, but I want to see how it will impact medicine."

For many involved in the medical field, the Barbadian experience of asthma necessitates a different kind of state approach than what biomedical research offers. When I asked one pharmacist whether he would like to see research into asthma, he responded, "I'd like to see the air clean. We need more education on environmental control, at least in the house." Others echoed this want for practical action over research. Polyclinic physician Jeremy Rowe similarly focused on a pragmatic surveillance: "I'm interested in seeing asthma clinics, asthma education groups, like we currently do with diabetes, and I'm looking forward to having something like that for asthma, for newly diagnosed asthma. We have bits and pieces of it. But not together." Several medical practitioners contrasted the biomedical research in Barbados with social research, often citing studies conducted on other diseases. For example, a pharmacist talked about dengue intervention that was attentive to the patient's daily practices:

They should probably be getting more involved in the education, and more *studies*. To find out what each patient have in common with each other. Like with dengue, you know dengue? They looked at what people have in *common*, environment, where the mosquitoes breed. They learn from when they actually *see* the person. So more studies, surveys, like that."

Such education and "social" research were frequently defined in explicit contrast to the numerous biomedical studies. One private doctor in the southern urban area, Nicholas Ryles, told me about social research on lifestyles. He continued:

I think this would give better information than the controlled studies. I think if you do a controlled study—a controlled study has specific guidelines, and you see how people come in and this is how they use their medication. There's a need for talking to the patients—it was done with diabetes care, by checking the number of times people were having their blood sugar tested, when they were actually seen by their doctors.

Nicholas devalued biomedical studies in Barbados for underemphasizing the experiences and practices of the patients. However, he went on to talk about the expansion of genetic research into asthma and other conditions. Given this direction, he hopes for the result of more objective techniques of diagnosing asthma: "I would like to see…the use of more scientific means, more scientific markers by introducing more measurement gadgets, more objective things. At this point, asthma is not like hypertension, not like with diabetes." This interest in genetics as potentially producing a more unequivocal, scientific diagnostic was common among general practitioners in particular, who often criticized the variability in diagnosis at the hospital, among the polyclinics, and in private practices. In the context of a widespread focus on biomedical outcomes, these practitioners hope for some standardization of techniques. An uneasy tension persists between a want for more "social" research and a valorization of the technologies brought by international biomedicine.

Skepticism about the research playing a role in Barbadian medical care did not preclude affirmation of genetics in general as the direction of biomedical research. One doctor who expressed doubt about the relevance of asthma genetics to treatment remarked, "Genetics is very important for cancer. I'm not sure about asthma, but genome mapping is the way to go." The inevitability of genetic research as the medical future was averred by almost all in the medical field.

Among the physicians and nurses involved in the genetics studies, I was surprised to find that this inertia of genomics research was not an accolade but a dilemma. One facilitator had a tone of resignation when talking with me about the increasing medical genetic research in Barbados and elsewhere as a part of modernization that was overwhelming in its complexity: "This genetics and genomics research. It's just going to go on and on." Physicians and nurses at different levels of study facilitation—recruiting patients, providing access to biological samples and records, administering research—gave a sense of their involvement in a massive project with a logic independent of Barbadian realities. They expressed varied criticisms of the research that they facilitated.

This plurality of views on genetic research was present even at the highest levels of Barbadian researchers, those who are coauthors on genetics papers published in peer-reviewed journals. I interviewed one doctor—involved in two genetics studies and a clear proponent of such research—in his office in an urban area. He remarked, "Genetics is important for asthma, but we are only scratching the surface. And for atopy. We haven't really got a firm grasp in the genetic area." This cautious enthusiasm was not shared by another physician, Lawrence Beecher, who provided participants from his private practice for a genetics study: "In terms of the asthma condition, when the first study was done twenty-three years ago, there was a 1.03 percent prevalence. This increased to 18 percent then 20 percent as found in ISAAC. Genetics does not account for the dramatic change." This emphasis on the incongruence between genetic research and the rising outbreak of cases was shared by many specialists and participant families, as I explore in chapter 6: several expressed doubt about the role of genetics, current or potential, in medical practice. Lawrence also considered genetic research unresponsive to the economic realities of the country; he went on to discuss the lack of facilities for genotyping in Barbados: "There's no place for genetic testing here; we had to send all of our work to Europe for testing." For Lawrence, the focus on genes and high technology makes the study inapplicable to Barbados, producing future treatments that will be restricted to wealthier countries.

However, he countered this image of uselessness in a later discussion we had on the potential significance of genetics:

> In terms of possible uses of genetics in asthma, there are the studies showing the genetics of non-response to antileukotrienes, and this leads to them saying, "Well, maybe that explains our patients who don't respond to beclomethasone" [a steroid inhaler]. And there are possibly different types of asthma. Genetics would be very useful in defining asthma—now, we have no objective means, as you know. We have wheezing.

Lawrence simultaneously criticized the nonutility of the study while valuing the potential of such research as possible correction to the contingencies of diagnosis found in Barbadian medical practice.

Another doctor involved in a genetics study described a similar ambivalence toward the motives of the international research occurring in Barbados:

> A lot of studies are being done. People are getting on the bandwagon, and studies are being done where drug companies give money to show their drug is better. And there's the genetic study. What I want to know is, how is this going to affect the way I treat the patient there [indicates examination room]? If there's no impact on what I do with the patient, then genetics of asthma studies are just for *Nature* and *Science* articles.

For this facilitator, the pharmaceutical company and academic interests are tied together in international projects that are in danger of being inapplicable to Barbados. This physician shared Lawrence's view that Barbados would be unlikely to utilize genetic technologies in medical practice.

As with the public officials described in chapter 2, this perception places Barbados into a global process oriented toward the future of medicine. However, unlike the state members, the study facilitators do not convey the sense that Barbados is making some use of this global process through its inclusion in international research; physicians and nurses involved in genetics projects considered the studies to be benefiting the goals of genetics teams or the interests of pharmaceutical companies. Such analyses turn the scale of projects from an asset into a criticism, implying that these global practices come from market interests. For these facilitators, the research integrates Barbados in the medical future and is simultaneously inapplicable to Barbados. The country's participation was left considerably more ambiguous in these accounts than in the public officials' perspectives. This mix of desire and skepticism toward genetic studies reflected the sense of a genetic future likely to leave the marginalized country behind. The speed and scale of genetics in these narratives was not a fecundity but a problematic excess. Such ambivalence creates deeply conflicted attempts to bring the research into Barbadian medicine.

Environment-Gene Interactions

Environment is a particularly openended medical category around asthma: most Bajan medical practitioners contrast the "environment" with household practices; to most geneticists, environment is everything nongenetic.

At the meeting between Taylor and the genetics-of-asthma group, Barbadian industrial practices were discussed. Taylor talked about the increase in dust at certain times of the year, relating it to roadwork and building construction: "I stress the prevention with my doctors, because there is more construction now. When you wash your car and set it outside and let the rain fall, it would look like you didn't wash your car. So we are breathing that right now." He went on to talk about a construction company near his house that caused dust. Other causes of asthma-related visits to the emergency room were raised, including Sahara dust (the allergens, smoke, and dirt brought to Barbados from Africa by winds) and the dust from cane harvesting (as Taylor put it, "During the crop season, the harvester spews dust about a mile high. The guys doing this can hardly see their eyes"). Through the genetics study, these causes, often discussed by Barbadian health care practitioners, are addressed. The collaborations are seen as bringing U.S. expertise to the particularities of Barbados asthma, placing the environment in interaction with genes.

The genetics group was particularly interested in the environmental aspects of asthma in Barbados. In Mary Warner's presentation on the genetics of asthma, environment was defined as exposure to endotoxin (an allergen in bacteria associated with pets, vermin, livestock, dampness, and other household characteristics) that interacted with genes. She discussed the very high levels of exposure in Barbados that her study found. A particular genotype protects an individual against asthma around low levels of endotoxin, but may be detrimental around high levels of endotoxin, resulting in worse asthma. The researchers found a low prevalence of this genotype among the Barbadian participants in the study, and concluded that this lack of protection may explain the high prevalence of asthma. Environment, as endotoxin exposure, is made an object in interaction with genetic background, and practices in Barbados, such as pet and chicken ownership and the presence of vermin, are analyzed with respect to the particular genetic variants found by asthma studies.

Through this depiction, genotyping technologies become critical to analyzing "environmental" causes of asthma. In a later presentation, Eric discussed different causes of the higher morbidity and mortality experienced by individuals living in poor urban areas in the United States. The environment that took shape in his narrative included tobacco smoke, ozone, and other air pollutants. Genetics in this talk was an amorphous influence: he depicted asthma as progressing from genetic predisposition to immune response, to inflammation, to wheezing. As Eric subsequently turned to interventions based on environmental research, genetics remained unspecified but significant among the causes of asthma. Eric discussed the differential morbidity and mortality from asthma in different populations as involving many nonenvironmental factors, and presented his own research into asthma severity employing genotyping technologies. The genetic research comprises the most extensive studies of allergens found in Barbados, and analyzing the environment—whether pollutants, household practices, or climate—here relies on genetic expertise and tools.

In the subsequent question-and-answer period, the Barbadian practitioner audience worked to make these findings relevant to Barbados's "environment." The physician/researcher Edward Wright asked whether the humidity in Barbados affected the kinds of pollutants that Barbadians would be exposed to, particularly in terms of the dust from Africa. This line of questioning—attempting to apply Eric's results to the specificity of Barbados—dominated the discussion. One doctor asked what particular interventions were employed in Eric's study—for example, how cigarette smoking was reduced, how contact with allergens was avoided. Another doctor wanted to know whether the intervention worked on both allergic and nonallergic types of asthmatics. Several questions focused not on the particulars of Eric's work, but instead appealed to his expertise. One doctor asked about the filters designed to reduce contact with air pollutants: "How effective are air purifiers? I have been telling my patients to invest in them." A similar focus on creating an intervention program for Barbados emerged in an impromptu talk Eric gave at the hospital to a group of nine physicians and nurses. He titled the talk "Is Asthma Increasing?" and discussed the complexities of determining levels of asthma and allergic conditions worldwide. When he finished, the first question asked was "What should we study here?"

The responses at both the conference and the talk left such specificity open: the humidity of Barbados was considered unlikely to affect pollutant contact; the air purifiers did affect pollutant contact but after nine months the effect on asthma attacks seemed to be lost; the difference between allergic and nonallergic asthmatics was not explored in the study. This ambiguity of results reflects commonly held views in medical research on asthma, as indicated in chapter 3. For the Barbadian doctors, these responses proved disappointing and frustrating in their desire to apply the international biomedical expertise and research to the Barbadian experience.

Environment is subtly reshaped through such exchanges. Health practitioners in Barbados implicate recent practices as environmental causes of asthma, including automobile use, modernization, diet, and building and road construction, as noted in chapter 4. This discourse is variably taken up by Barbadian researchers. One facilitator explained the causes of asthma in Barbados to me: "I think it is the pesticides and insecticides and chemicals. People use chemicals in their homes, everyone wants to use the strongest-smelling disinfectants. We see [families], they spray all over the kitchen."

These differing ideas of causes were used to doubt the interest in genetics. One Barbadian researcher remarked, "There are many studies. I'm still waiting to see if the information is useful from them. We need to know the effect of the environment on asthma, the wind, the allergen count, smoke." In a conversation with another study facilitator, I asked whether asthma was increasing. The facilitator replied:

> Yes, it seems like it. But I'm not sure. I mean, with all this research, but they still don't know [pauses] what causes it. I mean genetics is part, but there's got to be an environmental part too, doesn't there? I guess it's a lot of things. We eat different foods now; genetically modified foods are everywhere, aren't they, you don't even know if you're eating them. And industrialized countries are bringing all this stuff to places, saying they're making it better, but that's where asthma is going up.

For this facilitator, the international commerce that brings the genetics research in which the speaker takes part is implicated in the disease being studied.

The gene-environment dichotomy is thus ambiguously employed. Among many practitioners, the increase in asthma in Barbados is used to emphasize environmental factors and deemphasize genetics. As one Barbadian researcher involved in a genetics study put it, "There is a strong genetic disposition, but how much does the environment alter? Barbados is a closed unit, particularly on this island the genetic component is not going to change." Thus, the depiction of Barbados as genetically stable and homogeneous is used to direct attention to the Barbadian environmental experience. Environment is thereby contrastively and increasingly defined in opposition to genetics through the research. At times, medical practitioners reframe ideas of pollutants, dust, and pesticides as interacting with genetic predispositions, as they attempt to localize the research to the specificity of Barbados; at other times, they use this formulation of gene-environment to accentuate the lack of importance of genes to the Barbadian experience. For the Bajan facilitators, the research binary of genetic/environment creates new ways of formulating the effect of modernization and diet, requiring arcane knowledge and technologies that threaten to make the whole endeavor pointless.

Placing Barbadian Race into Medicine

Like environment, race takes on new significance through the international genetic research in Barbados. As mentioned, race is critical to all of the projects occurring there. The population is commonly cited as 92 percent black, and study participants are considered biologically equivalent to African Americans and other populations "of African descent." This percentage comes from the Barbadian census, which offers the following categories to mark for "ethnic origin": black, white, Chinese, East Indian, Arab, mixed, and other. In the 2000 census, 93 percent of those who responded marked black; 3.2 percent, white; 2.6 percent, mixed; and 1 percent, East Indian (Barbados Statistical Service 2002a). This classificatory system draws from common official designations of race in the English-speaking Caribbean (on these designations, see Khan 2004). The contrast of East Indian and white, or Chinese and black, reveals a relational nexus of race and nationality.[3] The national origins of Barbadians historically, aside from England and Africa, include, particularly, India (people imported for labor) and other Caribbean islands (particularly immigration from Guyana and St. Vincent and Grenada). (I discuss the significance of different racial identities among Bajan families in chapter 8.)

In the eyes of researchers and practitioners, Barbados is racially homogeneous. As asthma expert George Long put it, "There's not really a demographic difference here in Barbados, because it's so homogeneous, it's difficult to separate. The vast majority are black." For Edward—the Barbadian researcher involved in several studies discussed in the previous chapter—the census was somewhat misrepresentative:

> According to the government census, Barbados is 92% black, four something percent white, and a small percentage of Asians. There are a small number who label themselves mixed. The truth is that many who are mixed label themselves black. The North American political culture has made the description of black popular because North American tradition has historically been prejudiced against racially mixed people, so people are identifying themselves as black.

Edward, like many, places race as a historically and socially contingent identification ("label") while naturalizing a biological race ("many who are mixed"). His interpretation contrasts the census and other kinds of self-identification with biomedical realities. He continued: "In medicine, a popular definition of race and ethnicity is the majority of grandparents a person has, so if they have three black grandparents, then he is black. If a person has three Asian grandparents, he is Asian. And if he has three white grandparents, he is white. So there is probably an overestimation of blacks in the census." Edward, like most practitioners, thereby gives final authority on race to medical meanings, in contrast to either state statistics or self-identification. This approach of medically relevant race dovetails with the emphasis by genetics researchers on the moral significance of the biology of race and disease.

The research teams work to convey the value of a racial database to Barbadian officials and facilitators. During the conference presentation on acute lung injury (ALI), the speaker noted that the acute lung injury DNA bank includes Caucasians and African Americans. He remarked, "African Americans have a worse time with ALI than Caucasians. They have higher morbidity and mortality. This is why we are particularly attentive to ethnic-specific susceptibilities." The link made between Barbadians and African Americans as black populations is here part of making the moral case for the genetic research: the research is necessary as acting on the disparities that connect people of African descent. A similar sense of immediacy was expressed in the presentation on obstructive sleep apnea (OSA). After discussing the high levels of undiagnosed sleep apnea that are estimated to exist, the researcher talked about the problems associated with the condition (e.g., motor vehicle accidents, hypertension, and short-term memory loss). These medical effects were linked to ethnicity through the "increased prevalence of OSA in non-white populations" including Hispanic and Americans of African descent. Ethnicity was discussed as one of the risk factors for the condition, making Barbados a particularly important site of research. Later, the researcher made this link by noting that African Americans and people of African Caribbean descent with hypertension are at increased risk of stroke. In this representation, international biomedical research that ties divergent populations together as biological races is a necessary medical practice. Genetic research is framed as an urgent science (as in chapter 1).

Barbadian involvement is portrayed as a boon to this science. In Mary's presentation, she talked about the genetic significance of Barbadians being of African descent, referring to the common view discussed in chapter 1 that African populations have more genetic variation than populations in any other geographic area. This is taken to be an advantage for medical research attempting to narrow a genetic region associated with a medical outcome. Referring to the Barbadian research, Mary mentioned that "populations of African descent allow us to genotype fewer SNPs," making them "of tremendous value to the scientific community."

Barbados's contribution to this medical science creates new medical histories, linking black populations. For instance, Mary presented results that the genotype for more severe asthma is more common in black populations than white populations. She remarked, "The frequency of [the genotype considered to result in worse asthma around high levels of endotoxin] is low in African Americans and Barbadians, so we hypothesize that there is some selective advantage that made high levels [of an alternative genotype] for African Americans and Barbadians." She later noted, "We want to do a correlation of endotoxin with new concrete homes....So the disparities in asthma morbidity and mortality between different ethnicities we think can't be explained by environmental factors alone."

Mary's use of "selective advantage" refers to the ways evolution is at times used to speculate on ethnic histories: the results of the asthma study are interpreted to mean that African Americans and Barbadians, as populations of African descent, share a possible history of high exposure to parasites and diseases, and consequently the alternative variant—which protects against worse asthma around high endotoxin levels—was evolutionarily advantageous. These surmised ethnic histories are comprised in the nosology of the genetics of disease. Health disparities are understood to make genomic research among these populations critical.

These presentations of the moral immediacy of biological race-disease research create techniques around health and ethnicity in Barbados. Vague links of biological race and disease generate speculation about other conditions. During the question-and-answer period, one Barbadian doctor linked ethnicity and obesity as risk factors for obstructive sleep apnea: "Between whites and nonwhites, we also know in the U.S. nonwhites have a higher level of obesity." This physician wondered whether the triad of ethnicity, obesity, and obstructive sleep apnea might be biologically based. In a follow-up question, a Barbadian researcher asked, "In view of the ethnic data from North America, here we have such a high prevalence of obesity in women. Three times greater than that of men. Do you think it might be part of our metabolic syndrome?" Through these interactions, biologies of race were linked to emerging health trends in Barbados for the Barbadian physician audience, as the metabolic syndrome makes obesity, hypertension, and diabetes genetically linked to race. Prevalent illnesses become racialized and vaguely genetic in this process. In my conversation with Edward, he referred to the cancer genetics study: "There is a higher incidence of prostate cancer in blacks. This has been found among African Americans in the U.S., in Brazil, and in Trinidad and Tobago. So it is the most important cancer in black men." For Edward, as for others, this medical urgency is the primary reason for the need for studies of Barbadians that connect them with other black populations. Another Barbadian researcher explained to me the significance of the asthma genetics research by pointing out, "Blacks have more atopy and more asthma." The urgency of genetic research becomes part of medical logics as diseases take on racial and genetic significance.

Opaque Medicine

Medical categories of environment, race, and asthma are thereby realigned. To see how these connections are forged, I focus on what happens to a particular explanation for asthma through the genetic research. The "hygiene hypothesis" is one of the predominant explanations of the increase in asthma in different parts of the world among the international biomedical and epidemiological community. According to this model, modernization has led to decreasing exposure to infections and bacteria (we are raised in more hygienic environments than in previous times); as a consequence, our immune systems are more likely to react severely when we come in contact with allergens, resulting in more cases of asthma and other kinds of allergic conditions.[4] Part of the work done by the Johns Hopkins team explores the genetic expression that results in immune system response and the team is therefore examining the hygiene hypothesis in Barbados.

The Barbadian researchers I talked with frequently discussed this model, which most had learned about through international conferences on asthma in Barbados or from the asthma genetics studies themselves. The link between genetics and the hygiene hypothesis for these researchers is tenuous and often unclear. After returning to the office from a home visit, one Barbadian facilitator asked a Johns Hopkins geneticist about the results of the asthma genetics studies. (In the following exchange, "p-gram-negative bacteria" is an allergen that causes asthma attacks.):

RACHEL: Have you found a gene for asthma?

GENETICIST: There are many involved. In my work I found that the gene for the receptor for the p-gram-negative bacteria is connected with asthma. It's actually complicated because more receptors for the p-gram-negative endotoxin to bind to makes the person upregulate that part of the immune response which means they downregulate the asthma response. So, having the gene for more receptors makes you have less severe asthma.

RACHEL: Explain again.

After the geneticist did so, Rachel responded with the reason that she had asked the question: "Then, so, because the patients ask me what we're looking for." Mark, another facilitator, joined in here: "Yeah, that's the first thing they ask." The geneticist replied, "Yes, and but the reason that I haven't been telling them is that if they have the gene, then more dust will help them, so it's hard to know what to tell them." Mark responded, "So it's a balance."

Through such exchanges Rachel and Mark came to associate the gene vaguely with dust in the home and to see genetic research as particularly opaque. A link between the hygiene hypothesis and genes was both substantiated and entirely arcane: increased cleanliness was associated with genetic background in a way that required genetic knowledge to understand or utilize. Genetics thereby was associated with the forefront of biomedicine and centrally involved in asthma, giving shape to environmental and other explanations, in a way not usable to the Barbadian facilitators.

The hygiene hypothesis was also tied to race. In the conversation between the geneticist and Mark and Rachel, the geneticist talked about the ethnic significance of the results: "and, we found that the gene is exactly 50 percent less among African Americans. And the same with Afro-Caribbeans. So people of African descent have exactly half the chance of having the gene for less severe asthma." For the Barbadian researchers, an environment of exposure to allergens and household practices interacts with a vague genetic background associated with being black. These gene, race, environment, and disease interactions are knowable through international genetic research, as one facilitator indicated when talking about the various studies occurring in Barbados: "There's the cancer study,... the diabetes study, and there was the glaucoma study, also by Stony Brook, an eleven-year study. They did find that it was genetic—it's a black person's disease."

Diagnosing Genetics

These interactions reveal that new meanings of disease, ethnicity, and environment produced by medical partnerships have a dynamic quality, as expertise is diversely evaluated. Even as genes for asthma are revealed, the strangeness of "STAT6" creates an enigma for the Barbadian physicians that is only resolvable via high-throughput genotyping technologies. "Environment" shifts from being causative to being part of the background, from being demographic to being individualized, from a classification of industrial and agricultural pollutants to a set of household behaviors and livestock ownership. Race is linked to asthma through genetic results. Barbadian medical practitioners associate asthma genetics with the expertise, technologies, and scale of international biomedicine. For many, such research is simultaneously inapplicable, market-driven, misguided, and authoritative. This discordance results in frustrated attempts to apply the team expertise to Barbadian patients, creating new medical links, including asthma as opaquely associated with genetic background and various conditions as possibly "black person's diseases." These links are understood to require genotyping technologies in order to fully grasp them. At the same time, many practitioners want to make use of this problematic force of genetic biomedicine that will be the future.

Thus "illness" and "ethnicity" take shape through medical partnerships of Barbadian doctors and U.S. genetics teams, a shape that incorporates the technological and monetary disparities between the two, as well as the simultaneously valued and denigrated utility of genetic research. James Boon (1982: 121) notes that cultural meanings are not so much shared as exchanged. And I would add that meanings, like gifts, when exchanged are infused with the significance accorded the giver. For the Barbadian doctors, the genetic basis of race-asthma links is associated with U.S. expertise and the biomedical future: two associations that connote both authority and absurdity. These conflicting attitudes are produced between U.S. and British medical institutions and practitioners in postcolonial countries that provide patient populations.

With the extension of biomedical research into resource-poor countries, this genetic futurism is changing government policies and medical practice. Research "often anticipates a future it claims to produce," as Boon writes of rituals generally (1990: 124). As biomedical meanings of race and disease extend across national boundaries, postcolonial governments redefine the way their populations are racialized, and see illnesses as vaguely genetic. The moral discourse of the genetic future of race medicine gives a sense of urgency to partaking in the global market in medical research. This cultural life of utopics suggests the foundational contradictions by which biomedical discourses of race and disease are giving shape to current formulations of the state, illness, and ethnicity.

Chapter 6

Misgivings in Medical Participation

Participation in the asthma genetics study involves allowing the genetics team or facilitators into the home to draw blood from all family members, collect dust samples, and conduct questionnaires, allergen skin prick tests, and a spirometry test. Because the study is longitudinal and extends into other areas (e.g., asthma severity), this process is repeated over the course of years. The families that comprise the participant population in the study thereby accept a host of technologies and medical practices into their domestic space. In the next few chapters, I explore why, and what participation generates for the families.

What brings the families to the study? They are offered a small sum of money as recompense, but none of the participants I interacted with was particularly interested in this: often families were unaware they were to be paid until they received a check after the home visit, and none mentioned money in describing participation. To learn about the institutional and family practices involved in this participation, I moved from the home to the doctor's office, the emergency room, the pharmacy, the school, and roadside, to hear families of asthmatics talk about pharmaceuticals, agricultural policies, food importation, environmental hazards, medicine consumption, and single motherhood.

The meanings ascribed to biomedical diagnoses and prescriptions by families incorporate domestic economies and cycles of employment in

Barbados as in other parts of the world (see Das and Das 2007). João Biehl (2004b) interrelates the experience of biomedical categories with the determinations through which possibilities of life are shaped. He tracks the subjectivity produced in this nexus to question the concept of "medicalization" of individuals, making such identities more complex. Following such anthropological work, I attend here to the material conditions and political economies of care experienced by families, along with their more unstable and multivalent interpretations of these configurations (on such openendedness in the use of genetic results, see Rapp 1999 and 2003).

Troubled Categorization

Newspaper and radio accounts, medical and pharmaceutical attention, and public and private outreach programs have made asthma an object of public discourse. Today, almost everyone in Barbados has a family member or friend diagnosed with asthma, an opinion about the causes, and concerns about the prevalence. As one mother of two asthmatics told me:

> And when the parents come [to pick up her son for a birthday party] I would say, "Well, he has asthma."...Ninety-nine percent of the time, "Oh yeah, ours do too." So I wouldn't even have to send the inhalers. Because they have the—everybody has the stuff. That's how it is. Almost every person—every household has somebody in it with asthma.

This communal aspect confers a solidarity: as another mother told me, "It is everybody—everybody's disease." The dramatic increase in asthma is a consistent source of discussion, as I heard in medical contexts as well as in homes, on the street, and on the bus.

However, this increase was as contested among families as it was among medical practitioners. Katrina Moore is a participant mother of two asthmatics and is herself asthmatic. During an interview in her home with her children and husband at the table, she talked about the change in diagnosis:

> Now, they say it has increased a lot, but I'll be very honest with you. I have an opinion on that, and I think what has happened—I remember as a little girl when I was living here, there was always—Barbados had a cure for everything. If it went to the doctor. You sneeze, you cough, you wheeze, and it was wheezing, but nobody called it that. And I remember as a little child, I would—the noise that you make, what they called it is wheezing, that's what I used to do, right?...So, I think what used to happen is that people

had asthma. But nobody *recognized* it as asthma. Alright? There was no *name* put to it. And the people in the villages used their own remedies....So I don't know that it has necessarily *increased,* I think it was always there, it's just that we didn't have a handle on it the way we do now and everybody knows what it is now and you know, but kids always had these things! The asthma was always there. I always had the same, I had the same as Christian [her son] as a child growing up. And you know they rub you with this ointment, they give you this bush to drink. You know. So that's what I think. I could be wrong.

Katrina's reference to wheezing suggests the identifying characteristic for most Bajan practitioners. She was unusual in believing there had been no increase, but most families talked to me about the expansive diagnosis.

Some used this changing diagnosis to question the category of asthma. One asthmatic in her twenties indicated such uncertainty: "So I really find honestly that a lot of people who adult age are now being diagnosed with it, or coming down with the symptoms that could be characterized as asthma." Her narrative transition from "being diagnosed" to "symptoms that could be characterized" was an example of a prevalent opening of the category of asthma. These accounts separated the diagnosis from the experience, treating the former as one possible interpretation.

In this reflection on the diagnostic category, families expressed strong criticism of the medical techniques used. Leslie Foster is a participant mother of two asthmatics who lives with the children and their father, Steve, in an urban area.

> LESLIE: But like I was telling you that I was very sickly too when I was small. And at that time they didn't call it asthma but when I—my breathing to me is not a hundred percent. Because sometimes I be walking too and I just, find that I catching for air but yet still when I go to the doctor they said it's not *asthma.* It's not asthma, right. So I get short of breath a lot.
>
> AUTHOR: Did they say why they don't think it's asthma? What tests do they give you?
>
> LESLIE: They didn't do no tests! They just listen to my chest and stuff like that.

Leslie went on to criticize her medical designation as not asthmatic, a classification based on insufficient techniques in her view. The medical reliance on wheezing was particularly emphasized in such criticisms. During an interview with both Leslie and Steve in their home, Steve talked angrily about the lack of diagnostic techniques and attention in Barbados: "They don't do this thing! They just put them here on a nebulizer. Check them out every maybe half an hour. And then they're going to send the doctor over, as long as the wheezing has stopped, he gives you a prescription for medication and send you home." These families see a medical practice that uses wheezing pathologically: one mother remarked, laughing, "And do you know that as soon as they start wheezing, the doctor says it's asthma!" In their view, this myopic vision obscures the experience of asthma. Diane Boxer is an asthmatic in her twenties. I interviewed her and her asthmatic sister, Cathy, as well as their mother, in Diane's home. Diane recollected an event at the hospital:

> But I remember a time I had just came back from Puerto Rico, and I had a really bad infection....I remembered I was more having problems breathing and chest pains than actually *wheezing*. And I was trying to explain to the doctor—remember that Mommy?—And they couldn't understand that I was more having shortness of breath than wheezing! They were trying to say, "Well it's the wheezing that was causing it," but I could tell that it was more than just the wheezing, my chest felt like it was going to open up. But I guess they just sort of treat you for the wheezing part, but to me there's more to asthma than wheezing! They're too limited to that part, they always think, "Well you're wheezing so let's treat the wheezing part." But then, you go home, sometimes you got to go back down there! Because the main problem was not fixed.

For Diane, as for others, a compulsive focus on wheezing creates a frustrating diagnostic that precludes the patient from being heard.

This reliance on wheeze was particularly troubling for families, given doctors' willingness to unambiguously diagnose asthma. Cathy, Diane's sister, is a young asthmatic mother of an asthmatic. After telling me about the focus on wheeze among many doctors, she continued:

> And doctors are doctors, yes. Right? But I find that sometimes if you—they can only help you—I think they can help you best if they listen to what you *say* is going on with you....Because you can only know how you feel. And what is going on with you inside. They are just on the outside looking in. And sometimes they actually just diagnose and treat you according to what they *think* it might be, and they hardly ever listen to you! Just like in Diane's case where she had the infection from Puerto Rico. And she really needed to have that dealt with but they were just asthma, asthma, asthma. And that's what they were looking at! So I just believe that they should listen more to

patients about how they are feeling. And take it *seriously* into consideration. If they want to go ahead then and make their own assumptions, or their own diagnosis, that's fine. But definitely listen to the patient about it. Take the time to listen to the patient, and particularly when we talk to you, if they are in a situation where they can talk to you, listen to them.

Cathy here expressed frustration with the lack of voice experienced in the excessive certainty of asthma diagnoses, as various criteria are used to un-ambiguously categorize patients. Diagnostic techniques from "outside look-ing in" evoke the limited perspective of this different language.[1] This potent skepticism toward the medical diagnosis creates a space for assessing medi-cal advice.

The expression "doctors are doctors" revealed an opposition between patients and physicians common among the Bajan families I talked with. This logic rejected a medical hierarchy, instead posing different types of ex-perience and knowledge; both patients and doctors were expected to learn from each other.[2] Often, this criticism of medical practitioners included ignoring their diagnostic conclusions. One father of an asthmatic talked with the study facilitator during a home visit about his father being asth-matic even though the doctors said he was not. This man wanted his father to be involved in the genetics study, but his attempt was unsuccessful owing to the lack of a diagnosis. When I asked him later during an interview with him and his wife why he thought his father had asthma, he responded, "I know he is wheeze. I know he is wheeze. Always sort of [acts out labored breathing] wheezing." This man used wheeze as a diagnostic in opposition to medical practice, inverting Diane's criticism. But like Diane and others, he considered the problematic medical diagnosis to be incidental to the experience of particular conditions that involve difficulty breathing.

The potential asthmatic mentioned in chapter 4 is a common target of this skepticism toward the diagnosis. One mother I talked with at a phar-macy told me that she had brought her two children to a doctor for an un-related illness and that they both were incorrectly diagnosed with asthma; she used this experience to ridicule what she saw as the overdiagnosis of asthma in Barbados. For some, the study itself is the source of questionable diagnoses. Adele Campbell lives in an urban area with her asthmatic son. She does not describe herself as asthmatic, but she qualified this assertion during an interview in her home: "Well, I have never really had an attack but sometimes I wheeze, but based on the study I am an asthmatic. Within the study I am asthmatic. But I have never actually had an asthma attack. I don't recall ever having an asthma attack. But I know sometimes if I am sick, I will start to wheeze." For Adele, as for others, the study and medical practice both offer medical categories that are in some way arbitrary.

At times, such diagnoses were used to reframe past experiences. As in other instances when new techniques of diagnosis are introduced,[3] heredity was used to make meaning of events in family history, as in this account by a middle-aged asthmatic participant woman:

> You know, but now, well they get more—everybody studies and things. But they have people like—children they say are *born* with it.... They say it runs too with the heredity. Well see I have a brother from my father's side. And I never knew, I never put it to that—he died. And nobody never said—I never knew, but then when they find out that I was asthmatic, the girl said, "Well my daddy died, he had a, what we call a passover, but the night he died he had had an asthma attack!" And then I find out his grandchildren has asthma too! So apparently it came down from my father's side. You see?

Through participation in the study, heredity is made genetic and employed to retroactively make sense of family connections. Katrina talked about the causes of her asthma posed by medical practitioners: "They seem to think it's a gene that contributes to it. It's possible. Because even when I think back now, in my family so many of us must have had this thing, but we didn't call it that." Such genetic genealogies give new significance to "family histories."

This genetic asthma leads to ambiguous understandings, particularly in light of the increase in prevalence. The discordance between an emergent emphasis on heredity and the talk of dramatic increase results in conflicting accounts and unsure consumption of diagnosis. Lorraine Woodman is a participant mother with three asthmatic children. She expressed confusion about why there are more asthmatics: "And where did it come from?! I don't know! Because when you trace my family history, we are not asthmatic! You know? We don't have any asthmatics! But starting from my children, they all so with asthma. My brother has a daughter with asthma. Another brother with a daughter with asthma. And I don't know where it come from!" Lorraine's confusion and frustration revealed her distrust in heredity as an explanation of her children's illness, as she associated her experience with that of the community. The communal aspect of asthma, in which everyone is an asthmatic or has the possibility of becoming asthmatic, was central to the understanding of the condition for Barbadian families I met. The incongruence of this view with family-specific genes for asthma creates doubt.

The medical designation, in the eyes of these families, is one perspective among many to understanding their condition—a diagnosis that must be evaluated in the context of the perceived obsessive reliance on wheeze, the diagnosis of asymptomatic children, and the strange incongruities between heredity as explanation and the intense increase in numbers of asthmatics. And these questioned and questionable practices are inextricable from a perceived overemphasis on prescribing medications, for the families.

Consuming Medicines Skeptically

A diagnosis of asthma is inseparable from the prescription of pharmaceuticals in the accounts of families I talked with. They spoke alternately with humor, frustration, and knowing disbelief about the emphasis on inhalers among practitioners. Cathy talked about her experience with prescribed medications:

> I remember a time I was on—I can't remember all the names! Seriously, I was on so *many* medications....I know there was one that had—it was a little small glassy casing and it was green cover. Then there was one that was totally blue. Similar to Ventolin....Then there was one—I can't remember, I just remember the colors of them. And then there was one that was totally white. And it had a red cover. But I don't remember the names of the inhalers, to tell you the truth.

One asthmatic mother of several asthmatic children talked about being diagnosed: "As soon as I find out what it was, they give me the inhaler. And used to use the inhaler. They used to tell me take two puffs when you use the inhaler, something like that." The vagueness she expressed about how often she was expected to take the medication hints at her subsequent decision to discontinue use of the medicine, for herself and her children.

The families here criticized the role of the pharmaceutical in medical approaches to asthma. Patrice King is a young asthmatic woman who spoke particularly about this preoccupation during an interview:

> And I find people, as I said, people that I know of that have had one time occurrences of what we *assume* are asthma symptoms, and they will go and they were treated the very same way as a person who is *severely* asthmatic! And they are not put to the level where okay, this will never happen again, so I will treat you accordingly. Or this might happen again, so I will treat you

accordingly. They will treat everybody else the same, just because everybody seems to have the same symptoms. And give everybody the same things. So I think that somebody needs to do something about that.

For Patrice, the diagnosis and treatment reinforce each other's restricted scope. As discussed in chapter 4, among most medical practitioners, the link between asthma diagnosis and treatment is settled: the diagnosis leads to an unequivocal pharmaceutical. For the Barbadian asthmatics I talked with, on the other hand, the connection between treatment and illness is open, one where skepticism, modifications, and strategies are important. They criticized medical practice, therefore, not only out of a lack of trust in the diagnostic and prescription patterns they experience, but also from a perceived lack of critical analysis of the link between the two. I interviewed Hillary Randolph and her husband, two participants with an asthmatic son, in their home in a rural area. I had arrived soaking wet, having been surprised by a heavy rain as I walked to their home. I sat on the floor while Hillary and her husband sat in chairs and talked with me about their son's asthma. For the two of them, medical practice is unduly influenced by the focus on pharmaceuticals: doctors, lacking a more nuanced approach to diagnosis and care, are prescription writers. During a conversation about medical care, Hillary remarked, angrily, "They just, what I tell you, they just write the prescription up and give it to you." Her husband agreed, continuing, "I don't think the doctor knows. The doctors just want to give you the medication. They're going to give you what they look in their journal and see. Or they look in the journal and check the medication for you and give you that. And if you want to know anything else, you got to check your own doctor's book, or whatever." Cathy talked about this focus on medication with a sense of the absurd in her voice, during a conversation about a visit to the hospital for an attack:

AUTHOR: On that day that that happened, did they give you medicine?
CATHY: Yeah, the normal foolish Histal [an antihistamine] that doesn't work. [laughs] The Histal that doesn't work and then the normal—Amoxo— what do you call them—
DIANE: Amoxicillin [an antibiotic].
CATHY: Amoxicillin, which is the norm, so your body has it *so* much that it doesn't respond. Even when I was pregnant and I had to go to the hospital, I was about four months pregnant and I was wheezing for a whole week, and I went to there and they give me the Histal, and the *steroids* as usual. And I wouldn't stop wheezing so...

The view that pharmaceuticals are one treatment among many results in a doubtful view of the doctor's practice, as it tightly links diagnosis and prescription, without explanation or discussion of other causes and treatments. These families criticize the commercialized medicine based on the pharmaceutical by undermining the medical diagnoses and prescriptions they encounter.

In this perceived reliance on pharmaceuticals, patients expect from the doctor only medication; when this medication varies between doctors, patients see the need for their own intervention. This personal responsibility was particularly salient around side effects. Most of the asthmatics, and virtually every parent of an asthmatic, expressed a fear of the side effects of the inhaled corticosteroids. As discussed in chapter 4, physicians generally do not explain side effects to patients, arguing that doing so will only confuse them and further hinder adherence.

Every patient I talked with mentioned this lack of information from doctors. Cathy and Diane talked about this dearth in reference to the oral steroid:

CATHY: But the thing is with those medications though, the doctors—I don't know if it is the doctors, or is it the pharmacist—but you don't know about the side effects. The reactions. Because I remember I had read in a book about those same prednisolone [an oral steroid], the steroids, the things that cause the—they can, what is it now, the part about damaged, what is that part that leads to diabetes?—I can't remember the part of the body. But there are things that they can actually do to your body that can damage your body, but you are just given medication. But I guess we Bajans too we don't normally inquire, that is our problem, but there are side effects that you wouldn't—

DIANE: Unless it has the leaflet, then we would read it, but apart from that.

CATHY: But the side effects—but you are not told, you are given the medication and you're normally not told that this might happen.

Families spoke angrily about learning of side effects from other sources. Celia Hunt is a participant mother of three asthmatics. During an interview in her home, she spoke with increasing frustration in her voice about the lack of information on side effects:

I feel they should give a lot more information to parents. Explain things a little better. Especially at the polyclinic and at the hospital. About the medicine, the asthma, the side effects, stuff like that there. Because it was the Pediapred [a liquid oral steroid for children] they were using first, right? And it's only because their auntie in the states she got the information for me. And then a girlfriend called me and told me to don't give them because the certain side effects that they have but they never told me that!

As parents look to other sources—friends, books on health, alternative-medicine storeowners—they come across descriptions of drug effects that are often reason for ending consumption. During the interview with Leslie and Steve, Leslie explained:

> Because I basically don't want her to use the inhalers. If she live to see twenty-five and if she start to carry the cost and her bones are getting weak. They also said—and not at the hospital!—that we should try to keep more calcium in her diet. To keep building her bones. And her doctor never mentioned that to us! So other places that we go we hear things that can help.

The desire to avoid having pharmaceuticals in the body was not restricted to a generalized understanding that side effects exist and are suspiciously not mentioned by a doctor, nurse, or pharmacist. Asthmatics talked about many kinds of negative experiences from the medication, including brittle bones, joint aches, and racing heart. These experiences and the medical silence about them were particularly potent when asthmatic parents had to decide whether to give their children medications. For example, one mother remarked about the inhaled steroids, "When I take the steroids I get a lot of *pains* in my body. The doctor tell me it was strange, but I get *pains* and I can't sleep, and I cry and it has me—it's awful." Rose Wilson is a young participant mother of asthmatics. In one interview in her home, she fed her baby from a bottle while her other children sat on a couch, and she talked about her medical decisions as a parent. She described the reason she took her children off of their inhaled steroid in terms of how the inhalers made her feel: "I trembling, they got me trembling a lot. They make me tremble and help me feel nervous. And the medication that you go for at the hospital when you done get it, your heart *racing* so fast. And you can't stand up properly. To me it's got you *so* nervous." This effect made Rose wary of giving the drug to her children. Instead she gave them the older treatment of garlic water.

For many parents, the silence about side effects in the medical setting makes rumors and evidence of such effects suggestive of a dangerous secrecy. Two asthmatic mothers told me that at times the pharmacists at the hospital and polyclinic removed the pharmaceutical insert before giving them the medication. Ashley Williams is a particularly highly educated, middle-aged participant mother with an asthmatic son and daughter. During an interview she talked about such an event and saw a deception in this act that implied severe side effects: "*What* are they hiding from you?!...At the hospital, the pharmacist take them out. And I wonder sometimes why they take them out!...So that is something that I am a bit concerned about."

This sense of secrecy, of hidden negative characteristics of the medications that are being given to their children, produces fears and conjecture. These concerns largely draw from stories from families, Internet or medical book research, and an emergent influx of alternative-medicine literature and remedies coming primarily from England and Canada. The discourse on side effects is complemented by stories that circulate of asthma being caused by other pharmaceuticals. (Recent medical research on antibiotics has joined this chorus.[4]) One participant woman believed she may have become asthmatic because of an injection for paralysis in her hands. A participant mother of two asthmatics believed that her daughter became asthmatic owing to a pain medication she was given before undergoing surgery. The strategic silence around side effects is thus deeply implicated in the supposedly irrational fears around inhaled steroids. The pharmaceuticalization of medical practice is rejoined by these conjectures about medications and anger toward the practitioner's exclusive focus on diagnosis and prescription.

Interpreting Treatment

For the patients and families I interacted with, the perceived problematic prescription and diagnostic patterns of physicians and nurses are analyzed and tinkered with, but very rarely discarded. Within the political economy of health care difficulties, responsibilities of the family as caregiver, and the comparatively large funding and expertise deployed around asthma medications and diagnoses, families use the treatments they critique. Rose continued to feel ambivalent about her decision to have her children stop taking their inhaler:

> She don't take it [the inhaled steroid]. But she does still wheeze, like she was wheezing last month. Last month she was wheezing and so on, but I didn't give her the inhalers because, as I say, I don't want to put her back upon it. I know that *one* day we going to put them back on it, because asthma is something that can kill you, and you always have to have an inhaler. Because

I took myself off of it, and I was off for about four years or more....Because the doctor was telling me that even though I giving them the garlic water, some day they will got to walk with the inhaler or—it's a choice, let them die or walk with the inhaler. So I don't want them to die, even though they are so hard [laughs]. I would prefer to give them the inhaler. I be very skeptical, I will use my remedy first before I try to put them on the inhaler, because I think that weakens the heart. I feel it weakens the heart.

Rose here must contend with the doctor's warning of her children's possible death alongside her fears about unknown side effects. Henrietta Gayle, an elderly asthmatic woman who is particularly knowledgeable about asthma and medications, expressed a similar mix of distrust and use. During an interview in her home, she talked about her doctor's tendency to prescribe: "But I think Dr. Lander just changing things around, because these just come on the market. It was this—it was this one come on—Oxis [a long-acting β2 agonist inhaler], they advertised this just the last time....Then he give me this. So I just tell him, 'Don't give me anymore.'" Henrietta had previously talked about her asthma as being under control. I asked her why then her doctor had wanted to prescribe the new medication. She responded, "It just is a new product. Every time they have a thing about a new product. So I guess he just give me, you know, so I take it and try it." For Henrietta, skepticism toward her doctor's excitement about new products does not preclude consumption of prescriptions, but instead allows a tinkering with these practices, making frustrating and inadequate systems manageable.

These doubtful consumption practices include taking other kinds of treatments, particularly those associated with Bajan tradition, including bush teas, lizard soup, and garlic water. Bush teas are the most common non-pharmacy treatment, used primarily by the older generation. Often, these remedies are explicitly posed in binary contrast to the prescribed pharmaceuticals. Maria Carver is a participant mother of an asthmatic daughter. During one interview in her home in an urban area, she contrasted pharmaceuticals with older treatments; after telling me about the medications prescribed by the doctors, she continued:

Yes, when they give many things I will go and look and find out what it *really* good for, or what the effects! I just don't really take things and use something—my husband just tell me go use something else—I just don't take anything like that! And tell the truth, okay the person have a cold, and the doctor going to prescribe this medicine for the child, I don't give them often!

I don't give them all off! Because I don't like all these things in the system. In the body! As I said I will make my own bush teas. Some old folks would know what to give, and they would just pick the bush for me. Put them out to dry, wash them out good, and boil them and bottle it. And it is bitter, and she is cry, but I tell her is for her own good and she just drunk up. And I give her a little honey to take the taste out of her mouth. The bush tea is good. And it not only just for the cold, but also it will clean you out. And any other system, any other thing, body, any problem you have, it will help clean you out.

Here the knowledge from tradition is posed against the unknown side effects of pharmaceuticals. "Traditional" medications, in this sense, are not restricted to homemade remedies: blood or nerve tonics purchased over the counter at pharmacies are combined with honeys, or teas, or soups, or other remedies that have been learned from grandparents. These mixes never included a pharmaceutical asthma treatment in my experience, a reflection of the ways that biomedical techniques and objects are maintained on a different register from even other pharmacy-purchased remedies.

The posing of these traditional treatments in opposition to pharmaceuticals recasts the meaning given to both. As inhaled steroids and Ventolin have increasingly entered the market and medical practice in Barbados, older remedies have been symbolically transformed into "alternative treatments," with the attendant current literatures about alternative medicine playing a role in some cases. Katrina Moore, who talked earlier about shifting asthma diagnoses, used these older treatments to criticize the American commoditization:

The older people knew the bush for everything. Quite frankly a lot of the bushes that they boil are in a lot of the medicines that we use today. Alright? And they knew every bush and what was for what, and, you know....Because even when he [her son] was little and I would—the older people that live around here, they would say, "Oh give him this and give him that" but I was always very skeptical, right, but a lot of the stuff did work. At least treated the symptoms. And as I got older and I read more, I realized a lot of the—like the aloe vera plant which for years we knew in the Caribbean was a healing thing and now enough in America it's a bit, all this aloe, commercialized, it's the same aloe vera plant!

In such accounts, remedies remembered from childhood are reinterpreted when read about in current British and American alternative health books, recasting pharmaceuticals associated with commercialization. Distinctions of local/global and traditional/modern are here deeply relational.[5] As each side takes shape in contrast to the other, current imported blood tonics purchased at the pharmacy and the literature imported by the alternative-medicine industry can become local. (And as I argue later about oral steroids, so can the pharmaceutical.)

Pharmaceuticals in this interpretation—categorized as dangerous, of hidden or unknown effect, tied to marketing and problematic medical care—are consumed in contradictory ways. The process of taking and inhaling or swallowing (or refusing to inhale or swallow) asthma treatments prescribed by the doctor is a translation of medical meanings and practices. The Barbadian families who accept the prescription are accepting some part of the biomedical system of categorization, giving some authority to it, while at the same time—by determining when and how they consume the prescription—placing a part of it under their jurisdiction, appropriating it, making it their decision and practice. For the families, such consumption of biomedical techniques and objects mediates the distinction between biomedical and market discourses and more personal perspectives.

This mediation is typified by the social role of the pharmacist. In interviews with families and with pharmacists, pharmacies acted as a marketplace. An informal economy in medications exists through these stores. As discussed, asthma medications are officially free to citizens who have a prescription at participating pharmacies; in practice, they vary in their degree and periods of participation. Owing to difficulties in getting reimbursed by the government, many pharmacies at times charge for asthma medications. This practice, conjoined with the frequent problem of the polyclinic pharmacies lacking sufficient stock of medications, results in almost all of the families I talked with occasionally having to pay for asthma medications. Additionally, in order to avoid the fear and dangers of waiting until their child has an attack to get treatment, mothers of asthmatics try to get the medication without a prescription. Almost every local pharmacist will sell the reliever inhalers ($\beta 2$ agonists) over the counter, a gesture laden with the morality of recognizing the barriers to health care access, familiarity with a longtime customer, and acknowledgment of the market forces of competing pharmacies that will offer the medication for sale if this one does not. The pharmacy thereby becomes a site where meanings of disease, treatment, and pharmaceuticals are negotiated and exchanged, producing its own rationality of medical care.

Families use this space to produce a personalized attention, in ways identified by anthropologists elsewhere (see Whyte et al. 2002: 79–103). The pharmacist becomes a purveyor, medical caregiver, and confidant. Many parents talked about a particular pharmacist who was the most helpful with their or their children's asthma, as did this mother of three asthmatics: "The pharmacists will talk to you about [the medicines] and tell you if it is good and maybe educate you on how to use it and that sort of thing." The pharmacist was valued for this attention over the physician. Many used these interactions to give shape to the illness, as Maria described for her daughter: "Like if she has a cold or something and I go to the doctor, I will go and ask the pharmacist if he—describe her symptom to the pharmacist, and okay, they will go and mix whatever, their little own medicine, and they will give me." In this negotiation, the pharmacist becomes a source of medical knowledge that is constituted relationally for the patient, in an open-ended way that they find lacking in interactions with physicians in the public health care system. Owing to this willingness to exchange, the individual ostensibly most linked to the denigrated pharmaceutical is the medical caregiver most trusted.

Pharmaceuticals can take on unexpected significance in this context where they represent government intervention, medical commercialization, and mediation between biomedical and familial approaches to disease. The use of oral steroids particularly exemplifies this plurality. In Barbados, oral steroids are anomalies. As an intervention for asthmatics, they are tied to the pharmaceuticalization of asthma that has occurred in recent years. For the pharmaceutical industry, they are a consistent problem because they compete with the newer patented pharmaceuticals, and considerable funding is expended in the attempt to replace them with inhaled steroids as the primary therapeutics for treating asthma. In the Accident and Emergency Department, they are the primary source of asthma care, given to everyone who comes in wheezing. In this role, patients associate oral steroids with the conflicting values they hold about the medical system: too eager to prescribe pharmaceuticals, to diagnose asthma, but also the primary source of medical help and effective treatment. Patients therefore accept the prescription for oral steroids, but then do not take them as prescribed. Instead, they hoard them in their home.[6] This collecting of unused medicines includes the significance of the gift (Mauss 1990). The medication use reflects meanings of social excess and debt: Barbadians talked about the responsibility of the government to supply free medications and the feeling of personal responsibility to make use of this service. The families also use oral steroids to resist the newer medications that they see as being over-prescribed by the medical establishment: here, the oral steroid valued elsewhere as a medicalized pharmaceutical is consumed as a means of resisting the pharmaceuticalization of asthma. Further, the oral steroid now becomes associated with the Barbadian past, with a time before the impact of international markets that brought the doctors' habit of overprescribing and the focus on daily medicine. The oral steroid is thus an object laden with values of citizenship, medicine, and markets in surprising ways, often inverting expectations. Anthropological attention to the multiple meanings of such anomalies provides a corrective to seeing individuals, societies, or families as simple reflections of our analyses of markets, power, and expertise by focusing on where such logics are at times reversed, played with, or undone.

This role of the pharmaceutical reveals the values and practices by which Bajans take part in the medical system discussed in earlier chapters. Through these moments of doubt and use, the families critique and make meaning of the pharmaceutical as public health intervention; of the state/industry system of care; and of biomedical concepts of asthma. The families wager this skepticism within the context of their experiences of vagaries of care and fears for their children's health, integrating critique with what is at stake in the daily experience of illness care.

Participation in the study is a response to this medical system, among many of the families. In reaction to the perceived narrow emphasis found in medical practice—the focus exclusively on the pharmaceutical and on wheeze—families look to the study for an expanded understanding of their children's condition. Frustration with the secrecy, dangers, and gaps they see in medical care makes them look for alternative ways of treating this condition, and the study is one such means—another way of mediating the distance between the arcane of biomedical expertise and familiar daily habits. This additional intervention is particularly valued as addressing an aspect of their children's condition left unexplained in government intervention: the causes of asthma.

Purities and Pollutants of Modernization

The industrialization and modernization occurring in Barbados are deeply implicated in the cause of asthma, for the families of asthmatics. Maureen Johnston is a participant mother who lives in a rural area that had recently had roads put in. She summarized the causes of the many cases of asthma in Barbados:

> But to me our atmosphere in Barbados is very, very dusty now. It wasn't like this before. Right. To me in recent years it is got very, very, very dusty.

And it wasn't like that always.... It's just *dusty*, and to me our atmosphere is polluted. It's not clean! And you driving behind vehicles that are making a lot of *smoke* and that sort of thing. And then I find that people don't watch what their children eat. So I think it's a mixture of diet, poor diet, because you know everything's fast food, fast food. And these drinks that got all the dyes in them and things, which I don't really buy. That is be like a treat in my house. You know mauby? You know Barbados mauby? I always have mauby syrup in my house. My children always drink that. Always, always, always. And then I think it's a mixture of that and our atmosphere. To me it's getting worse and worse.

Almost every Bajan family I talked with about asthma shared this emphasis on "dust." They felt that there is more dust in the air than when they were younger, that this contributes to the increase in asthma, and that this is a serious problem. Dust included exhaust from vehicles, roadwork particles, dirt, and smoke produced by other households burning refuse (a common practice). A multivalence in the meaning of "dust" allowed the term to be used by families of asthmatics to criticize modernization (understood as increased roadwork, manufacturing, and automobile use), community practices (neighbors burning trash, smoking cigarettes), and, by a few, global warming (which was perceived as the cause of the winds bringing African dust).

Ashley Williams talked about the link between industrialization and asthma:

The exhaust from the vehicles, then there's a lot of *manufacturing* going on, and then there are more houses to me than there are trees now. And I think that there has a lot to do with it because the *oxygen* buildup and things be less. That's what I believe. You can only speculate. But that is what I really believe. That it has a lot to do with it. Because we have a lot of factories now that we never had. Regardless of what you say, you're going to have exhaust, you got more vehicles on the road, and it's more exhaust in the atmosphere. The chemicals from the plants. And then like there is more buildings, so you got more cement particles in the atmosphere. All of that there contributes to it!

Almost every asthmatic I met viscerally talked about this unclean air; many described directly experiencing it in the body.

This dust, exhaust, dirty air was considered both the cause of immediate attacks and a more insidious pollutant increasing the number of children with asthma. Steve and Leslie talked angrily about the change outside and inside the home, which they believed caused their child to have asthma:

> STEVE: Dust in the carpet. You can see that that is dust there. It's just—you wipe off this, and in a matter of minutes it's like that again because of the frequent traffic.... It has increased, I would say about 90 percent! Because I remember times when you would hardly see a car sometimes.... It's pollution, there are so many cars.
>
> LESLIE: Especially the air, that's what affect whatever you do.

Steve linked this increase to the constant road construction work: "This is the *city*. And the houses are so close, as I said, the dust rates. *So* dust. *So* much dust! It is difficult to maintain around this sort of dust. There are people that are worse off anyhow." The increased highway and car use resulted in little difference in such narratives between rural and more urban families. Frank Lawrence is a participant father of an asthmatic. He and his wife, Alison, live with their son in the northern region of the country, far from the urban areas. During an interview with the couple, Frank remarked, "If you are in a traffic jam from the morning, you get that air, right? If you are in a traffic from the morning you get a lot of exhaust. Not *if*, you *will* be in a traffic jam, because the amount of cars upon the road now." Families talked forcefully about the need for government attention to this unclean air and the alarming increase in polluting activities. In these accounts, the unclean air of modernization produces new diseases like asthma, similar to what the environmental officials discussed in chapter 4. For the families, this consumption of foreign pollutants extends to broader dangers from modernized diets.

Consuming Modernization

Changes in food are considered the systemic cause of the high prevalence of asthma by almost every Barbadian not involved in health care that I talked with, regardless of socioeconomic background, whether asthmatic or not. As food importation has dramatically increased, families implicate the more processed foods and artificial ingredients in the Bajan experience of asthma.[7] As noted in chapter 4, a medical discourse in Barbados links asthma to artificial dyes in candies and snacks. Families extend this to include a critique of the change in food importation that implicates international commerce, Americanized farming, and the rejection of tradition.

Many see the high asthma prevalence as the result of eating foods that are overprocessed, as Maureen, who talked earlier about fast food, explained:

> [In the past] you would be eating ground provisions like yams and pota-toes and that sort of thing. And you grandmothers and things soon mix up enough things, like enough porridge and all that and *feed* you and that sort of thing. But now everything coming out of a *box*. Or a can. And you know people don't eat ground provisions like before.

This contrast between the processed imported foods and the former healthy foods grown and prepared by friends and family was common among middle-aged and older people I talked with. The younger parents and asth-matics shared the criticism of processed imports, but emphasized more re-cent correctives, including an advertising campaign in which local farmers label their products "100 percent Bajan." During an interview, Cathy and Diane had a conversation about the new consumption:

> DIANE: We had a lot of importations at one point.
> CATHY: Exactly. And all these additives and things, these preservatives and additives that you didn't get before.
> DIANE: We find, it is only now that you are getting this 100 percent Bajan campaign, whereas we are trying to eat stuff that we grow here and every-thing. And try to cut down on the amount that we import. A lot of our main supply of food was imported.
> CATHY: But it's still imported though!
> DIANE: Yeah, a bit of it still is.
> CATHY: And our 100 percent Bajan food is still going to have the chemicals!

Like many others, Diane symbolically linked the artificial and foreign with recent changes in Barbados brought by international trade. This distrust of importation carried an affirmation of the natural and local, associated with the past (and the current return to the past with "100 percent Bajan").

This influence of markets has also changed farming, in the views of these families. Celia Hunt talked about increasing pesticide use: "They spray the ground where the foods are for the cicadas and so on. They put enough spray in the foods. I think it is the food that making the children weak. More asthma and so on....And when they spray the cane, all of we be sick. All of we is be *wheezing*, I got to carry we to the hospital. So I think it is the foods." The asthmatics I spoke with contrasted this poisoning of the foods with previous times, as Maria indicated during an interview after I had eaten some food she had made:

> Because I mean food has deteriorated a lot. We don't get the nice ground provisions without any chemicals and all that. Everything we get is chemicals, chemicals, chemicals. Even this meat that we're eating. Chemicals. They doing things, even the bananas, all that to force them to ripe. So it could be something along that line!

Ashley assessed the market incentives that polluted the purity of older farming traditions:

> A lot of the things that you eat are not pure anymore!...The people treating the fields to get bigger yields. The chemicals coming from outside and they want bigger tomatoes, bigger carrots, so all these chemicals, the chickens, they bigger, they injecting them, all of that there contributes to it!...because when I coming I never had nothing so. So that got to be in the '70s, the '80s, and onward and I believe that you seeing an increase in asthma!

In these evaluations, market forces and the foreign are critiqued as bringing a poisonous modernization that causes asthma.

The participant families consistently invoked the United States as the source and pinnacle of the changes occurring through international markets. Several talked about Barbados as following the U.S. trends of diet, pesticide use, and car use. Kimberly Jameson, who talked about her children's genes earlier, in a later interview told me, "We used to rely more on fruit, whereas we do using a lot of stuff that manufactured....I find that Caribbean people are more Americanized." Frank is particularly knowledgeable about pesticide use, having worked in sugar cane fields. He and Alison talked with me about the link between international commerce and pesticide use. Frank explained why pesticide use has gone up:

> FRANK: Because it's easier work? It's easier work, right, for the people that do agriculture.
>
> ALISON: And they see what Americans doing, and do the same thing.
>
> FRANK: It's true.
>
> ALISON: And everyone saying that there's trouble, and everything U.S. do, people here is do.
>
> FRANK: Not really, I don't really blame the U.S. for that, right, because you getting it in Europe and all around. It is a way to produce food cheaper.

People looking to produce food cheaper. And faster. The turnover faster. You got to control the disease, and then the amount of chemicals that you're using to get the plants ready in a short space of time, right.[8]

For Frank, and for many others, the focus on speed and reducing cost in food trade is a naturalized force with its own logic and momentum. In their perspective, these trends bring chemicals, pesticides, and overprocessed foods that pollute Bajan health.

Frank continued:

Like a plantation over there. [long pause] What I saying is, right? I is work about two months around here and there's a plantation out there. Right now they has got people that is work around the clock. You got some chemicals only can work in the night. They don't work in sunlight. And they dress down—the amount of suit this white suit is the whole mask, like you are going into space, right? To put these chemicals to these same plants! Now the plants are going to have the chemicals, you understand? . . . It's tons of chemicals going into the ground there. And then they got this thing, it's called the mist that control the white fly. Something like, it's a blower, the chemical coming out but it coming out like a mist through the blower. It goes on your back like a backpack and this blower like blows leaves, it just to control white flies and a lot of things. So you spray that plantation in St. George, yeah, but you got other homes there and the whole big district below there! . . . so the wind drift and carry it right down here! So it going to affect people!

Many families talked about inhaling pesticides while walking by plantations or in their own homes. Some discussed individual cases they were aware of where chemicals or other hazardous materials were disposed of in wells or near crops. In a subsequent conversation, Frank rooted the pesticide problem in government regulation and U.S. sales practices:

Right, they got some chemical that banned in America. Right now you selling it to the Third World countries! And we getting it down here. And it bad. It *causing* cancer. *Causing* asthma and everything. And the government ain't policing it, ain't saying, "Well, look, if you ban this chemical, why you selling it to me?" So they using it down here. . . . My whole foundation treated with chlordane. And that was banned *years* ago in America! This house here now twenty years but I treat this here—before I knew that it was banned—with chlordane.[9]

These analyses of pollutants brought or enhanced by international markets implicate the United States and United Kingdom in asthma in Barbados.

Consumption practices reflect these critiques of foreign pollutants and markets. Families minimize eating of artificial dyes and colors, stop frying foods, avoid processed foods, and purchase "100 percent Bajan" products. Most attenuate these practices according to cost—for example, canned milk substitutes from New Zealand cost considerably less than fresh milk, and so were generally used by poorer families. Through the consumption of food, families of asthmatics claim some control over these nebulous processes of international markets and modernization, negotiating the perceived reliance on pharmaceutics by medical practitioners with their own experience. Progress and pesticide production and pollution are all naturalized, as inevitable, as outside Bajan accountability, possibility, open-endedness. The consumption of foods is an attempt to domesticate, to bring these practices into culture (in the sense Lévi-Strauss uses[10]). These problems of chemicals, pesticides, and manufactured food are often talked about in terms of Barbados being dependent on U.S. agricultural markets and production, creating a sense of the United States as a powerful and inevitable force on Barbados. For some participants, involvement in the study is a reversal of this dynamic—an attempt to use the expertise of this source of international pressure.

Genetic Doubts

Participation in the study—from recruitment through involvement and interpretation—drew on these experiences and reflections on medical commerce, state responsibility, and U.S. influence. Most of the recruiting was conducted through the Accident and Emergency Department of QEH. The primary focus of the genetics-of-asthma study was on sibling pairs who are asthmatic (in order to look for shared genetic propensities), with subsequent extension by recruiting as many family members related to these siblings as possible. The former head of the Accident and Emergency Department or one of the nurses usually asked parents of diagnosed asthmatics (an inclusion criterion) if they were interested in taking part in a study. Participation was consequently gendered, as particularly mothers of asthmatics were brought into the study because of their repeat visits to the Accident and Emergency Department for their children's asthma. Danielle Clifford, a mother of three asthmatics close in age, talked about how she became involved:

> There was a nurse at the hospital. Because I was at the hospital with Leroy on a Monday and by the Tuesday I was there with Sam, and by the Thursday I was there with James! And she says to me, "I been seeing you the whole week but with different children." I said to her, "Well, all three of them are asthmatic." So she said that there was a study going on and she thought that I should get involved.

This recruitment process involved use of QEH as a primary-care facility, thereby generally excluding particular economic and ethnic groups, as one hospital physician explained, "A lot of asthmatics who are white do not come here; they have their own nebulizers at home. It's [US$100] for a nebulizer. The question is, 'How often does this child wheeze?' If it only takes [US$1.50] to get here, then it doesn't make economic sense to get a nebulizer."

Some families were recruited elsewhere. One mother described becoming involved through her children's school after she had told their teacher about their asthma:

> So it was known in the school that he was asthmatic and they were brothers. So I think somehow it got around—they was known in the school so when the asthma—when they were doing the study, they contacted the schools to see about siblings and asthma. That's how they got Adrian and Isaac's name. That was in primary school. Because it was known, and a *lot* of kids at that school had asthma.

Other sites of initial recruitment included polyclinics and some private medical practices, as physician facilitators offered potential participants from their lists of patients. This multisited recruitment relied on the spread of talk about the condition, bringing the families to the study as a kind of care to remediate the difficulties of the asthma experience within the problematic care they feel they get.[11]

Once siblings became involved, the process of recruitment focused on including other family members—parents, grandparents, cousins, aunts, uncles, nephews, and nieces. Mothers and fathers assessed the study in deciding which family names and phone numbers to give to researchers. Often, participants identified with the study strongly enough to try to bring in unsolicited family members. In one home visit, the team arrived to find that a woman had decided to invite her asthmatic sister so that she could join the study. In other cases, participants expressed regret that siblings or nephews were overseas, and thus unable to be participants. One mother had a son in the military whom she described as severely asthmatic and she repeatedly talked with disappointment about his unavailability for the study, which she thought would help him. In these cases, the value of the study as a kind of care was acute. At other times, when participants were asked for the names and contact information of family members, they demurred or occasionally refused. Recruitment into the study followed these convoluted kinship dynamics, as family members assessed the care provided by the study amid domestic economies, emigration, and familial bonds.

After being recruited, families made the research significant to the asthmatic experience. At a general level, the study was valued as intervention on the crisis of the communal increase in asthma. The perceived rise in the numbers of babies wheezing and in older individuals suddenly getting asthma was talked about with alarm and concern, as urgently requiring research, as Maria described: "They could really go out and do a lot of searching to find out what really for true causing these things, and not only like children who is seven years old, nine years old, like some babies, sometimes a couple of weeks old!" Here again asthma was seen as a shared experience, where narratives from friends, coworkers, and acquaintances shaped the understanding of the disease rather than personal memory (I only came across one family whose first experience with asthma involved an infant wheezing or person over forty suddenly having an asthma attack). Research was considered important as a benefit to all of Barbados, as Maureen indicated:

> I think it [the genetics-of-asthma research] is a good idea. Because it seems as if we have a lot asthma in Barbados. And then you do have people that die from asthma attacks in Barbados. Maybe not often, but once in a while you will have. Actually, I—someone who went to school with me who died from an asthma attack in maybe about 2000. And to me it is something that people should not be *dying* from! But it happens!

For Maureen, the study generated hope for information to reach the community in ways that the existing medical system is not currently accomplishing. For many, this attention was a crucial voice in the silence about prevention. The sense among asthmatics that Barbadian medical practitioners focus exclusively on treatment resulted in a view that the genetics study fills an important gap of research into the cause of asthma. For these participants, the genetics study was paradoxically a rejoinder to biomedicalized care in Barbados.

Here, the genetic research had value particularly as foreign, coming from outside Barbados. One mother, after discussing the significance of the study being American, went on to talk about how important the research was:

> It's wonderful. Tremendous. It's great. It's good because a lot of people not only in Barbados but I think a lot of people in the Caribbean that have it. I'm from St. Kitts and I never heard my mom—my aunt say anybody comes with that *problem* down there, with *asthma*. And I said that is very strange....But Barbados full of a lot of it. *Full.* Many people I know die from that!

Lorraine Woodman, who earlier emphasized the strangeness of the increase in asthma, similarly emphasized the necessity of non-Bajan action:

> AUTHOR: What more would you like to see from the research?
> LORRAINE: I want to know really, what is asthma? You know I think that a lot of Bajans need to know what really *is* it. Where it come from. How you get it....Yes, they give you leaflets and all that. Some people might not even read them. We need someone to really educate us on really what it is and how serious it is and the *dangers.*

Lorraine saw the U.S.-based genetic research providing needed medical knowledge, a welcome redress to the narrow focus of pharmaceutical pamphlets. Many participants framed their participation in the study as bringing such outside knowledge to Barbados, filling gaps and problems in the Bajan system of knowledge and care around asthma. As Frank told me:

> Right now I feel that they're doing a good job in the amount of research that's going on....You get a lot of research as far as—the people that make the, I think it is, the Ventolin inhaler, they sponsored the last one. So you're getting some help in research from these sorts of people. So I feel you're getting some good research. Information is passing. But the information is something, that the government ain't really, apart from the Queen Elizabeth Hospital; you got to spread out your wings into the polyclinics....You got to make people more *aware.*

For Frank, the research helps fill the urgent need for education about asthma to reach the workplace, school, and churches, a kind of expanding expertise.

These participants used the study to identify with the United States as a source of medical knowledge and funding. In many contexts, the participants proudly identified themselves as Barbadian citizens: as part of their political and cultural identity, with pride in industry, with the high levels of education and literacy, as individuals with rights to medication and health care, as non-British. But identification with the study was often a form of being non-Barbadian, of disavowing the Barbadian state care, as being, in a way, more educated, better equipped to handle the sickness caused by external institutions and policies impinging on Barbados, of being singled out for care. This is not to suggest that association with the United States and biomedical techniques and expertise is intrinsically non-Barbadian. Caribbean national identities have often included a valued internationalism (e.g., being Bajan can be about being international). In the case of the genetics study, its foreign character was part of its value: being non-Barbadian was precisely what gave it authority for many families.

The families reach for the technologies and information of international biomedical research out of their experiences of misdiagnosis, contradictory causal explanations, and restrictive meanings of disease. They seek the perceived legitimacy of U.S.-based medical knowledge and investigation as a corrective to problematic prescriptions and classifications. But this search is not unambiguous: this interest in the study was accompanied by a surprisingly (to me) strong sense of doubt about the results. Many parents felt that the research is unlikely to generate results that can be utilized, as this father remarked: "I don't know if they can do something to help someone else. We would like to see [the result], but we wouldn't know what to do with it." Some strongly questioned the facilitators on what is being produced by the study, what medications will result, who will benefit. However, this wariness did not preclude a belief in, and acceptance of, the research.

James Boon (1999: 248) reminds us that belief "contains the kernel of its own doubt." For the Bajan participants I talked with, belief in the study is inextricable from this suspicion about its results. The value of the project for the participants is as intervention and attention in the space created by silence around pollution, food, prevention, and parenting of asthmatics. The skepticism occurs within the context of asthmatics who are on several different kinds of medications, and the uncertainties produced by inconsistencies of diagnosis, treatment, and access to care. The families thereby looked to the study for care and knowledge despite their uncertainty of what will come of it; they valued it despite being perplexed by perceived inconsistencies, such as a focus on family history amid the increase in the number of cases. The research for these families is a pinnacle of medical expertise. Bajan families considered the study authoritative (within the field of medicine), more adept and sophisticated than the family doctor, but still, like that doctor, having only one constricted perspective. Thus the mother quoted earlier could remark, "Within the study, I'm asthmatic." Such questioning acceptance of the research was common. As I discuss more fully in the next chapter, for the participants, the research exhibits the extremes of medicine: its ability to help categorize and intervene on their children, alongside the problems of medical narrowness. The study is at once an alternative to Bajan medical care and problematically associated with the narrow focus of Bajan medical practice, both valued and denigrated as foreign, as families make meaning of their medical, illness, and research experience. These families participate in biomedical research as a paradoxical response to the perceived biomedicalized practices around asthma, expressing deep irony and skepticism toward the new system of care in which they take part.

Chapter 7

Participant Mothers

Women are effectively the focal point for the genetics study: when children have an attack, the mother is usually the family member who takes them to the Accident and Emergency Department at the hospital for care, where recruitment into the study occurs. During subsequent enrollment, these women are also the primary source of getting extended family involved. In addition, during data collection, mothers are the ones who gather the family together for the home visits. I explore here how this gendered participation is significant for the mothers involved.

Medicalized Parenthood

Bajan participant families I talked with spoke often about fear as a critical part of the asthmatic experience. One woman vividly described getting an attack:

> Yes, yes, and you get like—and then your feet and everything. And by the time you going like this [acts out labored breathing], your *whole* chest *hurt* you and your shoulders....I have had it in the middle of the night since my husband died. I'm here *alone*....But sometimes you choking, you so, I catch myself just holding onto the bed and feeling—it is a prob—I don't even like to *imagine* it. You know?

This fear was similarly evoked by parents when talking about their children with asthma, particularly in the context of the suddenness of attacks and difficulty in reaching the hospital. Katrina, Christian's mother, talked about the constant danger of the condition:

> Christian will be sitting here, he'll be good. After like five minutes, he'll be like wheezing out like crazy! It just comes on—his comes on real *sudden.* So it scares you because one minute he is really good and the next minute—or he's outside playing and everything's fine, he's fine all day, and then he comes in and it's like [she makes a popping sound].

Several mothers talked about this immediacy, and their fear that their children might die from the condition. One mother of a teenage asthmatic told me, "To tell you the truth, at one time I would never think he would've got to the age of *ten,* as far as the age *sixteen.* It was really—it was bad when he was young." Involvement in the genetics study was partially an attempt to intervene on this frightening and dangerous unknown.

In these accounts, each mother's fear was based not only on her child's welfare but also on her own role of being medically responsible for the child. In Barbados, as elsewhere in the matrifocal Caribbean, women have historically been the heads of households. As Christine Barrow (1999) argues, family networks in this context tend to extend from the mother-child relationship more strongly than the man-woman one, which is frequently characterized as loose and unstable (for this reason, some have recommended the term "household" instead of "family" as more representative of Caribbean social life (Senior 1991)). Carla Freeman (2000) points out that in Barbados the female head of household is a symbol of strength and the perseverance of society while simultaneously having the least political economic power. Single motherhood is highly prevalent in Barbados: according to the 2000 census, 45 percent of women living with their children said they have never been or are no longer with a husband or common-law partner, and 45 percent said they have been or are (Barbados Statistical Service 2002a). Despite a long Bajan (and Caribbean) tradition of extended kin providing a social network, mothers told me that they relied very little on other family members in caring for their asthmatic children, except in the case of getting the child to the hospital during an attack. In the polyclinics, pharmacies, and at the hospital, I often saw grandmothers and aunts bringing asthmatic children in for treatment and getting prescriptions for them. As in other Caribbean households, these family members often lived in the home with the mother and child. Care of asthmatics is therefore often gendered to begin with, independent of the particularity of medical practices around asthma.

Mothers talked about this role of medical responsibility for the asthmatic child. As Maria Carver remarked, "And you will just see me always wipe off the chairs and the bed and you know, everything. I always work *hard.* I try to protect everybody, not only her alone, but everybody in here, you know." In this social identity, mothers become medical interpreters, learning to read the subtle signs particular to their children's condition. Maria talked about the initial diagnosis:

> One time, I never forget...she just had a little cough and I gave her some-
> thing, and then suddenly just saw her chest would go in and out, you know,
> like a drum. We call it "African drum." In and out, in and out, and I continue
> watching it and I said no. And so I rush her to the hospital and then they
> started describing it and they said, "Okay, she is it."

Sometimes this surveillance is achieved despite what the child says. During an interview with Leslie, she talked about needing to look for signs from her daughter underneath her words:

> Right when I look at her I see—"You stomach alright, you feeling well?" Be-
> cause she don't like to say no. She don't like to say when she is getting sick.
> But I can always look at her and see how she's breathing. I am accustomed to
> seeing her breathing because I monitor her a lot. So when I see she look con-
> cerned I say, "You're supposed to take your inhaler" and monitor her more
> closely.

Given the reliance on the emergency department for care, this ability to read their children was critical to mothers. Sharon Lorde is a participant mother of three asthmatics. She discussed this urgency around her daughter with me:

> Flora, she just have this cough and this sore throat and then she gets quiet.
> And she's not able to use anything. And then immediately she'll get like an
> attack. And we have to rush. Can't breathe, and she got this tightness, and
> the chest will be rising up and catching from breath and sometimes it's loud.
> Loud. Sometimes she scared us! Even the doctor was scared.

Like all difficult identities, this social role of responsibility for the asthmatic child is ambivalently meaningful: in this case a source of pride, frustration, weariness, pain, and strength (on such ambivalence in the social role of motherhood in the Caribbean, see Rowley 2002).

The evident gratification mothers expressed with their abilities was accompanied by fear when the children were in other contexts, outside of the domestic space. The school, a site to which the robust asthma intervention and detection program in the public health system does not extend, is an object of particularly strong fear and anger for mothers. Mothers spoke about teachers unaware of asthma signs and of the lack of medical staff there. A few thought that problems with school buildings caused the high asthma prevalence or attacks among children (a view also found among families in the United States). One mother with an asthmatic son and daughter close in age spoke emphatically:

> And every teacher that changes as the semester changes I let them know Marcus and Patrice are *asthmatic* and write it down on the *form* for the teacher to see! On all of their books, they have *asthmatic,* they bad *asthmatics!* In case that they say, "Look, I am not feeling well," at least the teacher could say, "Do you want to go home? Do you want to go the hospital? Do you want your mother to come for you?" You know? Because the doctor was telling me too that there's also—the nurse and the doctor—the silent one, whereby the lung, taken from the outside—let's say that your lungs be shutting off on the inside and you could die—you just lay down and say you ain't feeling good you could die that way too!

The unknown and possibly sudden ways to die from asthma make cryptic medical warning and school ignorance frightening issues that mothers are responsible for negotiating.

The schools, like other institutions, frequently placed accountability for the asthmatic with the mother: she is called if the child expresses concern about an oncoming attack, and she is often expected to bring the child to the hospital. Many women worked more than one job and relied on friends or family for transportation, making this responsibility particularly difficult.[1] As Celia remarked about schools:

> They need to educate and sometimes if a child is having an asthma attack, they will prefer to call me from my job. There's no one there really *trained* to deal with the situation, or until the ambulance get there, because it's now teachers in Barbados don't ever put your kid in their car to take them to the Hospital.... So they prefer me to come, or the ambulance.

Some mothers told stories of the school calling the mother before calling an ambulance when a child was having an attack. Leslie gave such an
account:

> A friend of mine was saying when her child took sick and before they called
> the ambulance to take the child to the hospital, they wait until the *mother*
> come there to call the ambulance! They should call the ambulance to carry
> the child to the hospital! Call the mother, right, the mother meet the child at
> the hospital. Asthma, you can see the child wheezing. Or take it upon your-
> self to get the child in the car and get the child to the hospital! You under-
> stand? Because sometimes there is not always an ambulance there! So you
> can see the child is wheezing—all of them got somebody, but they have to
> have a car. After the child get to the hospital, well. But the point is to get it
> there, because sometimes you get to the hospital it still ain't help. But at least
> you might get it *there*, you know you do your part. You don't just sit back and
> say, "Oh we got to wait for she, the mother come here, because the mother
> going to carry she to the hospital."

The reference to the ambulance is a common statement: ambulances frequently do not arrive in sufficient time, at times break down, or can take
hours to get the child to the hospital, according to both patients and medical practitioners, as noted in chapter 4. Mothers spoke with a sense of frustrated futility about this institutionalized deferral of responsibility.

This conferred duty often conflicts with work requirements. As many
have argued, motherhood and working for money are inextricably linked
ideals of womanhood in the Caribbean (Sutton and Makiesky-Barrow
1977; Massiah 1986; Senior 1991; Barrow 1999; Freeman 2000). In Barbados,
this work includes a mix of formal labor (wage work in services, manufacturing, and historically, the cane fields) and informal work (including
making clothes, jewelry, food, and other items to sell) (see Sutton and
Makiesky-Barrow 1977; Massiah 1986). Bajan women have increasingly entered wage work over the last forty years, partially as a result of the emigration of Bajan men to work in Canada, Britain, and the United States
(Barrow 1999; Freeman 2000; Safa 2005).[2] All the mothers I met worked
at least one job (e.g., childcare, construction, secretarial work), and many
supplemented their earnings with other ways of making money (selling
baked goods, sewing).

To reach their children when a school calls, mothers had to leave work,
with varying consequences: several mothers told stories of warnings or

reprimands from employers for particular instances of leaving to pick up their child (or to find a family member with a car to do so). Others said their employers were understanding. Most families agreed that employers will use the diagnosis to discriminate in hiring practices. Katrina talked about two of her work colleagues who hid the fact that they had asthma. She would bring her son's extra inhalers for them to use surreptitiously. During the interview with Leslie and Steve, Leslie talked about the necessity of hiding inhalers at work:

> If you tell people that you got asthma, nobody going to want to hire you. You understand me? Because they saying that you going to miss a lot of work. You ain't going to come to work because the asthma is affecting you. Anytime you going for a job interview you cannot let them people know that you have asthma! It's later on, when you get a certain way into this organization, then you can bring out your inhaler.

At this point Steve joined in:

> STEVE: But you want to take your inhaler. And you at your desk there and you want to take your inhaler, you take it out the desk there and going to get up and go to the bathroom and take your inhaler. You don't want nobody seeing you, right, you got to hide it.
> LESLIE: You got to hide that.

The institutionalized deferral of responsibility for the asthmatic to the mother is negotiated in these secretive practices (hidden inhalers) and angry denouncements of schools, workplaces, and medical facilities.

Filling Prescriptions, Responsibly

In addition to their role of reading the signs and getting their children to medical facilities during emergencies, mothers are given the role of medication facilitator. Obtaining medication includes evaluating contingencies of available time, money, and medical care. After making a diagnosis, physicians will invariably prescribe a medication, usually both reliever and preventer inhalers, which can be filled at the hospital or polyclinic pharmacies. After this initial prescription, the patient must return for another diagnosis in order to receive a refill. But the Accident and Emergency Department at the hospital will not prescribe medication unless the patient is currently having an acute attack, in an attempt to reduce the use of the department for primary care. Mothers who arrive with their children to obtain medication are told to go to a polyclinic. The polyclinics will prescribe the medication, but this requires several hours of waiting to see a doctor, owing to lack of funding—again a barrier that is often insurmountable because of workplace responsibilities.

These systematic difficulties are often experienced in conjunction with inconsistencies of care. As noted, in practice the polyclinics often run out of the medication. Parents and asthmatics related various difficulties encountered in the public medical facilities, including being told they could not come to a particular polyclinic and being given the wrong medication. This sense of capriciousness of the polyclinic made many parents extremely angry, a reaction that usually included fear: every parent I spoke with considered it dangerous to place responsibility for his or her child with the polyclinics. One father starkly remarked, "The polyclinics in Barbados is death traps. Medical care in the polyclinics, as far as asthmatics concerned, death."

Mothers gave accounts of contending with unpredictable responses at the polyclinics. As Celia related, "I took him there in the morning, and I said to the nurse, 'He was wheezing and I want him to see the doctor.' So she said to me, 'How do you know this child is wheezing?' I said because he's my child and it's not the first time he was in this condition. She said, 'But he does not look like this to me.'"

Adele Campbell told of being sent away without an inhaler:

Because I remember a time they didn't have the inhalers, so I went to—I took them to the polyclinic. I was *real* mad, because I took them to the polyclinic, that was the first time I have ever taken them to the polyclinic actually....And I asked the doctor to give me the inhalers because I don't have any more. He told me he can't give me the inhalers, I got to go back to the doctor that gave them the inhalers in the first place in the polyclinic to get the inhalers and when I went and tell the nurse, she was real *mad*. So then the evening she asked the doctor, and he wrote a prescription and I went for it the next day.

Adele drew attention to the personal aspect of her encounter with the doctor, as if she were being punished for her appearance or behavior. Her emphasis on the nurse's corroboration conferred medical legitimacy on her frustration, undermining the doctor's attempted hierarchy. Mothers in these moments appropriated their social position as medical caretakers of their children: they claimed authority as medical interpreters of their children's condition to rejoin attempts to invoke medical expertise.

These difficulties with the polyclinics are the primary reasons why the great majority of Barbadian asthmatics use the Accident and Emergency Department of the hospital for primary care; but there too mothers felt that their knowledge and needs were often not respected. An asthmatic woman talked about trying to get prescriptions refilled: "[After getting a prescription] you don't worry to run back up there before the month! Because you're not going to get it. Because they say, 'You waste it, you waste it.' Or 'You overuse it.'" Diane Boxer also talked about this adherence discourse at the hospital:

> I remember a time I was in the Asthma Bay and this doctor—the Asthma Bay was full and as soon as you—as soon as one person went, another one would come in, and I remember this doctor saying, "If the asthmatics—if they had took their inhaler properly, they wouldn't be in there." This is a general assumption, that you go to Asthma Bay, because you are not taking your medication *properly*. When we all know that most of the time when you see people at Asthma Bay because…the *coughing* gets *so* horrible, the medications ain't working, because your lungs are *still* closing! But then there's this general opinion from the doctors that okay, you are not taking your inhaler properly. This is wrong!

Diane here voiced a widely held critique of the adherence discourse that I talked about in chapter 4, as inattentive to the realities of the illness and medical experience.

In this space of fear, responsibility, and perceived lack of voice, mothers negotiated medical care for their children. When Steve and Leslie and I were discussing medications, Leslie related her attempt to get a refill on her prescription for a reliever inhaler:

> And sometimes, if I go to Queen Elizabeth Hospital I got to go to casualty the doctor will say, "Oh, the child ain't sick" and they can't prescribe the medicine unless the child is sick. I mean like if she's not sick but her medication runs out. And I say, "Well, I ain't waiting until she sick to get this medication. Let me go and ask him if I can get this medication."…So I go for them two [the reliever and preventer inhalers]. And the [reliever] Ventolin one when I go back, and the lady tell me, "Look, that here is supposed to last a month, so the month is not up we cannot give you a repeat." I say, "Look, but she using this every day. And it gone! And you have repeat on the box! So I come to get another one. I ain't going to just come and call for it and don't have one."

Steve interjected here: "Because she doesn't take it, she is not asthmatic! You know?" Leslie responded, "I tried to tell she that, but she say, 'No I can't have it, I have to wait!' " When she has the money, Leslie, like many others mothers I talked with, purchases the reliever medications in order to have them available. The mother-as-medication-administrator contends with medical hierarchies (e.g., by using pharmacists and nurses to gain authority that is suppressed in interactions with doctors) and institutional impediments (e.g., by relying on informal medication economies). Frustration with these processes reflects the lack of acknowledgement of these hardships.

Spaces of Expression

The mother's experiences around the asthmatic child—her fears, fatigue, employment difficulties, domestic labor, and medical facility barriers—have no institutionalized language. Mothers are medicalized only in relation to the asthmatic, not as themselves suffering, fearing, and laboring around asthma (on such dearth of institutional support for the social role of women in the Caribbean, see Rowley 2002). These experiences are discussed in personalized conversations with other parents, usually mothers, as I saw and was told by parents. As a result, the mother's experience is not only individualized but also made into a subjective experience for which she is responsible. The discursive silence around the role of mothers of asthmatics results in various ways of not acknowledging the pain of this role: deviations from the regimen, medical emergencies, and uncontrolled asthma are all in some sense made her responsibility, in a way that is not explicitly acknowledged (and therefore not discussed as a source of hardship). In medical facilities, I saw physicians repeatedly ask where the father was when women became angry for the sake of their children; nurses in interviews often criticized mothers for not understanding their child's medication; teachers talked with me about mothers' inability to discipline their children about using asthma as an excuse; and some physicians explained to me that women cared more about fashion than their children's health.

In this process, the register in which mothers express their anger and fear about the problems they face as caretakers of asthmatics is also individualized. Connections to other mothers of asthmatics or to the gendered space of the Accident and Emergency Department asthma area were rarely expressed. For Rose Wilson, the burden of sole responsibility for her children as asthmatics is linked to her own asthma:

> Because one day I was carrying three of them at one time! Three of them—
> Tanesha, Jonas, and Tyrone! And then when I get there they had to nebulize
> me as well, because being that I was thinking about them and their sickness

and so on, I too start wheezing. I was wheezing really bad. So it was real hectic and then I couldn't sleep. Had to be getting up checking them and so on. That is really scared me, because I say I am sick, they're sick. And I don't have anybody around to look after us, when I sick, so that is really scared me, it was real hectic. Sometimes all I could do is cry....My mom she would— if I feel sick now, my mom and them they'll help take care of them. But if I go work, I will take them there. But their father is not around and so on.... [One father] is in England, [the others] don't really come around as such. If Tyrone is sick and he could call and see how he is doing and so on, but he won't come. So it's just me and the...children. And it's really hectic.

Rose's misery and experiences implicate the social role of the mother of the asthmatic, gaps in health care that result in lack of ambulance access and routine medical attention, and economic shifts (which resulted in mass migration to other Caribbean islands and to England, as well as increased labor in the formal economic sector). Yet her expression of this misery was personal and individual, with a tone of despair in her voice. The mothers angrily denounce the inadequacies in health care and the school system, but the silence around the labor, fear, anger, and barriers they experience creates a noncommunal critique of the treatment of parents of asthmatics.

Personalized Medicine

The genetics study occurs within the context of these silences, anger, fear, and distrust. The hope generated for the study is to fill the space created by the lack of consistent and adequate medical attention and explanation. During home visits by the genetics group, mothers referred repeatedly to helping their asthmatic children and asked what would happen for their children from the study. This personal attention is affectively significant in the context of their largely individualized experiences.

For many, this is the most personalized medical attention they have received. Several participants explicitly linked their involvement in the study to their anger with the care they get, as did this mother:

Yeah, the—once, when she was very bad—the head doctor—because nobody be over a head doctor—the head doctor be over them—she was there but she was there like *dictating* to the about five trainees what is wrong with Cynthia [her daughter] or what should Cynthia do. And she didn't talk to me! All she said was, "I am doctor, and these are the trainees and I'm just running a session here." You know, and she say, "Oh, mommy, Cynthia will be okay," you know, that's it! And she don't take time to say, "Well, she'll get better," but as time get by, different people will advise us, you know, how to stop the asthma, try to avoid drinks with dye, and you get the literature about how they doing the asthma [genetics] study. We share with a different lady [from the study], not nurse Candice [a facilitator], and she explained to us how the breathing is supposed to be and stuff.

This woman went on to equate the study with the good medical care found in the United States and as an intervention on these Barbadian difficulties. The (implicit) gendered aspects of asthma care bring her to the study as a source of knowledge and attention to her concerns.

For some participants, the attention of the study itself is a kind of intervention. Lisa Sinclair, an asthmatic in her late twenties, talked with me about what she valued about the research:

To tell you the truth, it, I don't know, I see it as, like someone is actually, someone actually notice that you exert yourself as an asthma sufferer, and they want to get to, if they can, get to the root of your problem, or try to help you, or find ways that can help make your life easier for you as a asthma sufferer. Because all along before that you are just going along with this disease, just as you may be a cancer sufferer or HIV and you just go along with this thing, you know, and you're only given the attention from the physicians and the people that you might come in contact with when you're having an attack, and if they care, then they give you the attention. But the study to me, it literally pulls you out from the general population.

This is striking partially because Lisa is in a higher economic bracket than most of the participants, and sees a private doctor regularly of whom she speaks highly. Participants repeatedly expressed this sense of an intangible benefit from the attention and interactions with the researchers. One asthmatic mother of four asthmatic children, when I asked why she got involved in the study, told me how wonderful the researchers were, and that she liked being with them. These mothers valued participation as a form of extended attention, information, and care they miss in the state or private health care system, and consider the genetics team a medical authority that rejoins the dismissive Barbadian medical authority.

These family narratives show an involvement in genetic research premised on desires for foreign medical expertise to ameliorate the vagaries of Bajan care. The parents and asthmatics join the study to answer the unknown crisis of increasing asthma among family, neighbors, and friends;

to redress the inconsistencies and frustrations of public medical care; to feel a personalized attention amid the hostility of individualized and gendered medical responsibility; and to act on their child's precarious health. The sophisticated technology and focused attention of the research provides an identification with U.S. medical knowledge, as response to depersonalized medicine.

Chapter 8

Home Visit Translations

The following is a home visit experience reproduced from my field notes:

We walk up to a house made of wood and concrete, resting on cement blocks, with sheets draped over the windows as window shades. As we enter the home, a woman in her mid-thirties greets us kindly but with watchful eyes—"Good morning," she says. There are four of us: two Barbadian nurses who facilitate the genetics study, a student employee from Johns Hopkins University, and myself. As we enter, there are two mothers sitting at a table, and three children stop their playing to watch us. One of the nurses asks if there is a plug somewhere; after some rearranging of fans and couches, an outlet is found. The setting-up process involves laying out four glass tubes in which to collect blood, plugging in a vacuum cleaner with a special receptacle to collect dust samples, preparing a questionnaire with identification codes, and plugging in and booting up a computer connected to a spirometer, an instrument used to measure lung function. The two mothers closely watch the process with a look of suspicion, apprehension, and interest. When the tubes are laid on the table, one of the mother remarks, nervously, "That's a lot of blood." One of the nurses explains, "No, it's really not very much, just drink something beforehand, like a glass of orange juice, something with sugar." The woman nods absently and looks at the bottles. When the other nurse comes into the room after making a phone call outside, the mother again mentions her worries about the blood. He offers a similar response, attempting to allay these fears. She asks what will be done with the blood. The student employee replies, "We'll sequence the DNA." After a pause, she explains, "To compare to a person who doesn't have asthma, to see if a T is a C or something like that." The woman nods, says, "I need to see it written down, you know," and laughs. One of the study facilitators points out the consent form. The woman looks it over distractedly. The other woman asks, "What's the study for?" One of the nurses replies, "To find out what are the causes of asthma." The woman asks, "To find medicine?" One of the nurses replies, "Eventually, yes. First to find out what causes it." The woman nods.

The home visit usually began with a phone call to the participants, setting an approximate time for us to arrive. Locating the homes almost invariably included backtracking and circling, asking passerby for help, as we followed directions based on neighborhood landmarks because the roads had no signs. The homes of the participants varied but largely fell in the middle economic range of Barbados: they were often a mix of wood and concrete and usually in the process of being remodeled, according to a common practice of doing some work on the home with the intention of completing the work when more money becomes available. As a result, many homes stood on cinder blocks, awaiting the building of the foundation, and several had leaks that, during the rainy season, resulted in the children gathering containers to capture the rainwater dripping in. The tradition of extended family members living together often resulted in more than two adults living in the home, and in smaller homes sheets were used to partition off larger rooms for privacy. When we arrived, a mother of an asthmatic always greeted us. After introductions, a space was found or made for the team to work, including searching for an electrical outlet and a surface for the computer and blood tubes. The setting-up process then began.

The home visit is a cultural exchange requiring mutual translations, as the facilitators and genetics team gather data and samples, and the Bajan families make use of U.S. medical techniques and expertise. The genetics researchers turn the Bajan family meanings of ethnicity, wheezing, and illness experience into a science of race and disease. The Bajan families make the research team's technologies, descriptions of genes and asthma, and test results into meaningful ways of understanding their and their children's conditions. These exchanges reveal mutual evaluations of authority as technological and medical designations are created and used in ways that escape consistent representation.

Gathering Data

For the genetics team, the home visit is the process of data collection. This includes taking blood samples; administering the Adult Respiratory Health Questionnaire; conducting spirometry[1] by having the subject blow and inhale into a handheld instrument that is connected to a laptop computer; and vacuuming in various areas of the house to collect dust samples, including the mattresses, curtains, and pillows in the bedroom, living room, and kitchen. The questionnaire covers various aspects of asthma experience: history of wheezing, chest tightness, cough, breathlessness, medicine consumption, and so on. Other personal characteristics are also recorded, including height, weight, smoking history, and ethnicity. The genetics team uses these materials and data look for correlations between genetic regions; asthma prevalence (measured by physician diagnosis, methacholine response, patient description); severity (measured by number of visits to the emergency department, number of attacks, medication use, IgE levels); atopy (measured by skin prick tests, IgE levels, methacholine response); and environmental factors (including animal and cockroach dander).

Locating Asthma

The variable asthma classification discussed in chapter 3 is highly salient for the genetics team. One team member, Laura Stevens, talked with me about different genetic approaches to asthma during an interview in her office at Johns Hopkins. As she told me, clinicians disagree with epidemiologists about the cutoff point for what is asthma. She talked about the heterogeneity of techniques in different studies. Eric Reid echoed this sentiment during a discussion at the asthma study office in Barbados, joking, "To an immunologist, any wheeze or cough is asthma." He was particularly attentive to the ways asthma categorization has changed: he noted that determining the rate of increase of asthma in the United States is confounded by the change in questioning by the CDC in 1997. For the team, these competing definitions are a source of strength of the asthma studies: instead of relying on a single definition, the genetics studies in Barbados employ multiple methods to determining and measuring asthma.

Several different approaches to asthma and atopy are used in concert in the study: The respiratory health and asthma severity questionnaires ask about the patient's experience of wheeze, chest tightness, cough, and shortness of breath, at different times of the year and in general. Spirometry is used to measure lung function in reaction to an allergen or to a medication. A history of diagnosis by a doctor is requisite for inclusion. Atopy is also studied, through measurements of IgE levels and skin prick tests. The questionnaire and spirometry represent two techniques of asthma measurement, and are valued by the genetics team precisely in their contrast: The asthma questionnaire, based on patient history, is considered not susceptible to the problem of changes in asthmatic experience that affect spirometry and methacholine challenge. Conversely, spirometry is considered an objective measure in contrast to the possibly subjective measurement by the questionnaire. This method of several diagnostics and measurements confers an advantage over other asthma research in which single variables are used, in the perspective of the researchers.

All of these measures—contested in medical literatures—must be negotiated in study facilitation. One Johns Hopkins geneticist interpreted the spirometry results of the Barbados Asthma Genetics Study to indicate that the Study was poorly administered, resulting in underestimations of asthma severity, but later decided against this interpretation. A Barbadian researcher I interviewed explained his view to me that the methacholine challenge employed in the project was "useless as a measure of asthma." Diagnosis by a physician was opened to question during the conversation with the Barbadian facilitator discussed in chapter 5, in which Eric asked about competing diagnoses. This complexity is also found in the home visit interaction, where the meanings and experiences of the participant families must be translated.

The process of making these Bajan family experiences exchangeable with other biomedical definitions occurs primarily through the questionnaires and the spirometry technology. The spirometry computer program is used to record biometric indicators for lung function, including age, sex, height, weight, diagnosis of asthma, and measurements of lung capacity. The respiratory questionnaire, as discussed, categorizes asthma in terms of wheezing, shortness of breath, tightness in the chest, and cough. Of these, wheezing is the most commonly used to indicate asthma in medicine (and is also used for diagnosis by the International Study of Asthma and Allergies in Childhood). The responses to these questions required interpretation.

The contrasting emphases on time in the asthma experience exemplify this negotiation. Bajans talk about asthma more often in terms of seasons than months of the year. The questionnaires are particularly attentive to this distinction, dividing the year into summer, the rainy season, and Christmas break until Easter. However, the questionnaire and participant families place different emphases on the temporality of asthma. The study focus on how often asthma attacks occur, the number of emergency department visits per year, and when the first asthma attack occurred are not focal points for the Bajan participants. They emphasized the time spent at the hospital or the polyclinic, the duration of the attack, and different periods of treatment, whether pharmaceutical or otherwise. As a result, their answers to the questions about the first attack and number of visits to the emergency room were often vague or uncertain. The questionnaire includes the following directions for inquiring into asthma:

> Have you ever had asthma?
> If the subject does not know what asthma is, code as uncertain. If the respondent asks for more information about what is meant, say, "Asthma is an illness that generally lasts for more than a short time. People with asthma may have wheezing, cough, and shortness of breath, sometimes these symptoms come in attacks and sometimes they are always present. Would you say that you have asthma?"

This explanation separates the interviewers from the participant. During one home visit a mother diagnosed as asthmatic explained that she had "grown out of that" and that the questions about the symptoms (e.g., cough, tightness of chest) were not applicable to her. In another home visit, a mother deferred to the expertise of the team as to whether she had asthma. When the study facilitator asked, "Have you ever had asthma?" The mother responded, "No, please. Not to my knowledge." She was interested in whether the spirometry revealed her status. In these interactions, the significance of the research as a form of biomedical care and expertise for the parents becomes part of the interpretation of familial and scientific meanings.

Barbadian contestation over the diagnosis of asthma also arose in the study facilitation (as for the mother discussed in chapter 4 who found that she had asthma within the study despite not having had an attack). The participant who wanted his father involved in the study, mentioned in chapter 6, had the following exchange with the study facilitator:

> TERRENCE: My father, you can talk to him.
> FACILITATOR: He has asthma?
> TERRENCE: Well, I *think* he has asthma.
> TERRENCE'S WIFE: But the doctor said he doesn't.
> TERRENCE: Yeah, the doctor said he doesn't.
> FACILITATOR: Okay, well if he doesn't have asthma, if a doctor hasn't *diagnosed* him with asthma, he won't be in the study.

Terrence, like others, wanted to bring a family member into the genetics study as a form of care that he felt lacking in the Bajan health care system.

The researchers work to interpret these vernaculars of wheezing in stabilizing the definition of asthma for study.

The Home Environment

The concept of "environment" was similarly divergently settled by the researchers and participant families. The Barbados genetics studies present asthma incidence and severity as occurring through the interaction of multiple genes and environmental factors. For the researchers, the study transcends the limitations of purely genetic or purely environmental studies. Genes exist here in their ability to interact with known triggers, such as smoke, dust, and cockroach dander, and environment exists in its interaction with alleles associated with allergic response. This categorization requires the myriad complexities of Barbadian environmental meanings to be shaped in a way that can interact with the gene.

The asthma questionnaire focus on the home contrasts with the meaning of environment proffered by the Bajan families. In chapter 6, I discussed the latter: the roadwork, diet changes, insecticide sprays, and vehicle exhaust: pollutants brought by recent modernization. The questionnaire focuses instead on household behaviors that are thought to be related to asthma. This is not to suggest that the study instruments are inattentive to the particularities of the Bajan asthmatic experience; the questionnaires are quite sensitive to such specificity: for example, analysis of one questionnaire on household endotoxin exposure includes weighting for windows left open, recognizing the high level of endotoxin exposure from livestock around the house, often chickens, and grain handling. The study is thus highly attuned to Bajan household practices based on more than a decade of work in the country. But this emphasis on household is divergent from the ways the Bajan families interpret asthma causes, as seen in chapter 6. This considerably different focus often resulted in the lack of clear responses, as in this conversation:

FACILITATOR: Did your mom smoke when you were a baby?
MOTHER: I don't know.
FACILITATOR: Your dad?
MOTHER: I don't know.
FACILITATOR: To the best of your knowledge, how much did you weigh at birth?
MOTHER: I ain't sure. [laughs] To tell you the truth, I ain't sure.

FACILITATOR: Were you breast-fed by your mom?
MOTHER: I don't know those things! If she was alive I could probably find out.

These behavioral factors were not part of the repertoire for understanding asthma for the Bajan families. Their unimportance to the families usually necessitated several exchanges as facilitators attempted to make differentiations and designations out of their absence among family members. The reciprocal process was also highly visible during home visits, as families attempted to designate practices undifferentiated by the study. As the above questionnaire administration continued, the mother's emphasis on causes of asthma emerged:

> FACILITATOR: [Do you wheeze] when you are exposed to chemicals, like strong perfumes, hairsprays, insecticides?
> MOTHER: Yes, dust.
> FACILITATOR: Dust, which we already did.
> MOTHER: And certain things like at work, chemicals, that is make me sneeze a lot!
> FACILITATOR: Yeah, that went under chemicals.

The woman then told a story about being at work and the particular chemicals in use that made her unable to breathe and forced her to sit down. The genetic research classifies such work environments, chemicals in the air, and construction materials with household practices, such as use of hairsprays and perfumes. "Environmental" causes of asthma transform from the pollution of global commerce to the household background.

This transformation allowed participant concepts of "environment" to be stabilized in interaction with genes. The research team found the presence of pets and carpeting to result in more exposure to house dust, as other asthma research has found. The team places these practices into interaction with gene expression, resulting in a new understanding of the hygiene hypothesis, linking modernization and development with genetic susceptibilities of particular populations. At other times, the genetics team interprets the complexity of the environment as noise—a set of confounding factors that make the causal effect of genes undetectable—resulting in the inability to precisely locate the low-level influence of a genetic predisposition to asthma. In order to be placed in interaction with alleles, the environment is translated: dust as roadwork, pollution, housing demographics, and living arrangements are transformed into IgE levels, or the presence of gram-negative bacteria. The families and researchers both posit a modernization in explaining asthma; but where the families look to pesticides, artificial foods, and exhaust—these market pollutants—the team looks to changing household habits, a domestic modernity.

Stabilizing Race

Race must also be translated. As noted in chapter 5, geneticists represent Barbadians as biologically black, identified with African Americans. For the genetics team, this link is forged by the research in two ways: first, through self-identification as Afro-Caribbean on the questionnaire, and second, through analysis concluding that Barbadians are genetically similar to African Americans.

Race in Barbados, as elsewhere, is multivalent. My explorations of race/ethnicity among Barbadians was marginal and I offer the following as pointing to some of the complexity of the interlinked meanings of race, ethnicity, and nationality in Barbados, rather than a systematic account. As anthropologists and historians exploring ethnicity have shown, ideas of class, race, gender, and religion interweave unpredictably in discourses distinguishing others.[2]

In my conversations with Bajans, the dichotomy of black and white, the strongest racial contrast in Barbados, was talked about particularly historically with reference to colonialism and class difference amid the current control of major industries by white owners (as discussed in Beckles 1990). I was occasionally told about the shift toward black identity as coming out of the political developments of the 1960s and 1970s (as other analyses of race in the Caribbean have discussed, e.g., see Harrison 1995; Robotham 1996; Hall 1997). This identification as black involved a historical association with Africa, and an expressed link with U.S., British, and Caribbean black peoples.[3]

But the various nationalities represented in Barbados are also inscribed in meanings of race. Indian, Guyanese, Chinese, white, and Bajan are all contrasted with each other at different points. Thus, while "black" is used to describe race, the meanings accorded to race/ethnicity preclude an easy juxtaposition of white/black from the United States to Barbados. Katrina Moore explained races in Barbados in contrast to those in other Caribbean countries:

In Trinidad, there are a mix of races, East Indian, black, Asian, and so on. But here they don't mix. You won't see East Indian mix with black. In Barbados, there's white and black and East Indian. They came over before the black people as indentured servants, so they are native Barbadians. But the East Indians stay with the East Indians. And when they watch cricket, they watch East India. If you see black people with a mix, it's Guyanese.

Races and the level of distinction between them were differentiated by nation, as anthropologists working in the eastern Caribbean have explored (see Yelvington 1993; for subtle discussions of the ways claims of heterogeneity and hybridity are constituted in Trinidad, see Khan 1993 and 2004 and Segal 1993).[4] This view of races as more distinct in Barbados than in other Caribbean countries was routine among the people I met, particularly in opposition to Guyana (as is common in the Caribbean—see Maurer 2000). Guyanese immigrants, as the largest Bajan population born in another country, both represent and trouble this distinction.

Racial/ethnic distinctions here operate at different levels, at times delineating black from white (politically, economically, culturally), in other cases Chinese from East Indians, and at other times Bajans from Guyanese. Race and nationality were occasionally discussed as reinforcing each other. In talking about the different races of Barbados, several Bajans explained that they could identify the difference between Caribbean nationalities based on how the person looked. One mother remarked on this scrutiny as it was applied to her: "I have lived in Barbados all my life. I know persons normally look at us and ask if we are Bajans. And we hardly have the name here. We are Carver. They hardly have that name here, so I don't know if our ancestors from somewhere else. I don't know. I have never researched it." Surnames were often used as markers of identification. In talking about family background, two study participants had the following conversation:

DAUGHTER: Our great grandfather from my father's side he was a Guyanese. But from what I know the others are Barbadian. Mommy, tell us what our foreparent background? From your side was?...Daddy's great—daddy's grandfather was a Guyanese.

MOTHER: Oh! Uh-huh, Uh-huh.

DAUGHTER: Part Vincentian because our name. Our surname....Okay, well, it was only Guyanese from my great grandfather's side.

Name, nationality, ethnicity, and race were thus interlinked and used contextually to identify distinctions.[5]

These moments of contradictory identity are critical to ethnic/racial meanings. Racial identities are a means of exploring, pronouncing, and playing with otherness. Ritual spaces designed to explore this contradictory space are found in Barbados as elsewhere, as in the national holiday of Crop-Over. Crop-Over is by turns considered the Bajan Carnival and posed explicitly in contrast to Carnival, as clothing, dance styles, skin color, moral behaviors, geographic ancestry, tradition, and ethnic background are all identified in contrast to those of neighboring countries.[6] The relational aspect of social categorization, including race—always about a border, a boundary, that is, about some other group—is explored in these spaces. Such multiplicity reveals not categorical chaos, but rather the lack of consistency of culturally rich codes.

In the home visit, these contradictions interact with those of a genetics of race and disease. The different focus of the study—on race/ethnicity as a biological category—results in a classification system that precludes nationality. The Barbados Asthma Genetics Study has two areas in which the study facilitator marks race. First, the spirometry software has a category for ethnic group, following the shift in U.S. biomedicine replacing the use of race with ethnicity. The options are Caucasian, Afro-American, Mexican American, and other; under other is listed Afro-Caribbean, which is the category the study facilitators use. The software also includes the option of ethnicity in order to adjust the lung function results for ethnicity, under a category marked "Ethnic correction (%)," but this section was not used during study facilitation (see Braun 2005 for a subtle discussion of the history of this technique).[7]

The other area for racial categorization in the study is the questionnaire, which asks:

The following is necessary for genetic purposes:
Is your racial/ethnic background:

Afro-Caribbean
Caucasian
East Indian
Other
If 'Other,' specify

The questionnaire goes on to ask the racial/ethnic background of the person's mother and father, with the same options for response—as noted, a common method in medical meanings of race, in which parental race is used to categorize the participant. For example, in the Collaborative Study on the Genetics of Asthma (CSGA), "Ethnicity was self-reported, and in families with mixed racial parentage (less than 10 percent of the study population), the race of the proband was specified as African American if at least one parent was African American and Hispanic if at least one parent was Hispanic" (Lester et al. 2001). These two systems of racial designation—parental and self-identification—come into contact in the home visit, where the participant families and study facilitators translated such meanings.

During the questionnaire administration, the facilitators would usually phrase the question as "What is your racial background?" or "Is your racial background Afro-Caribbean?" dispensing with listing the options. Responses to these questions varied, incorporating the complexities of racial identities listed earlier; the study facilitator interpreted the responses, as in this case:

FACILITATOR: Is your racial background Afro-Caribbean?
MOTHER: Beg your pardon?
FACILITATOR: Your racial background, your race.
MOTHER: Okay, Caribbean.
FACILITATOR: Yeah, Afro-Caribbean. And your mom and your dad the same, yeah? [Mother nods]

Identification with the Caribbean was thereby turned into a biological link in these interactions, through questions largely considered perfunctory. The more common response by families mentioned being black or African (e.g., "We are African," or "Black, of course, no maybes about it").

Several responded with indications of nationality, drawing from the contrasts discussed earlier. One woman answered the question about her parents' racial background by saying, "My grandmother is Portuguese." Another responded, "Father and mother both from Guyana." One mother who identified herself as Bajan commented, "Well, to be honest with you, my grandfather was white. But he married into black....So we came down that line. But my foreparents were white." In these responses, the Bajan families emphasized relational meanings of ethnicity, drawing together Caribbean heterogeneity and family histories, with a sense of multiple solidarities. In response to a question I asked about parental background, one mother remarked, "They are Bajans. Bajan." Her husband interjected, "Bajans, Africans." The mother responded, "I don't know. I go through my mother. My mother and father Bajans," and laughed. This multiplicity—contrasting a solidarity with Bajans, a history with Africa, family affinities, and humor about this multiplicity—is critical to identities of ethnicity. What was particularly intriguing was the degree to which individuals created a pause in these assertions about race to the researchers: a hesitation was evident in the statements about not having that name here, and white foreparents, and Bajans as Africans versus as Bajans. In these pauses, the families expressed the discrepancy between the liveliness of ethnic identities and the stability of an identification inscribed for medical analysis. Their sense of the researchers' desire for such stability could thereby become a part of the study.

The study marks these responses as Afro-Caribbean. In the shift to data analysis and presentation, the meanings of race employed in the Barbados census are translated into the meanings from the U.S. census. For the genetics team, the basis for this transformation from Afro-Caribbean to African American is genetic.

The genetics team argues that both African Americans and Barbadians have approximately 25 percent Caucasian admixture, a percentage employed in articles and conversations. This datum is based on an analysis conducted by some of the team members in collaboration with another group of geneticists, examining the prevalence of a gene involved in the expression of a blood group protein (DARC) (Nickel et al. 1999). Individuals who express the protein are called Duffy-positive, and those who do not are Duffy-negative. Other biomedical research has found a very low prevalence of Duffy-positive individuals in West Africa, and genotyping of a different allele (Fy^a) involved in DARC expression has been used to analyze Caucasian admixture (Graves 2001: 201–3). In the present study, individuals were genotyped for two alleles (DARC −46C and −46T): homozygotes for DARC −46C are Duffy-negative, while those who have at least one −46T allele are Duffy-positive. The results were produced from three primary populations: 90 individuals chosen from 33 families in the Barbados asthma study; 93 individuals from a population in Cartagena in Colombia; and 235 individuals from 126 African American families participating in the CSGA, recruited in Chicago, Baltimore, and Minnesota (644 individuals) in addition to 48 African American individuals from the University of Chicago. The analysis found that Duffy-positive individuals comprised 35.74 percent of the African Americans and 21.11 percent of the Barbadians. This result is interpreted to indicate an approximately equivalent Caucasian admixture between Afro-Caribbeans and African Americans.

As discussed in chapter 1, biomedical uses of race are multiple, drawing on sets of genes, attribution by skin color, self-identification based on census categories, and geographic location. When biomedical researchers enter neighborhoods, homes, and doctors' offices, they come across other sets of distinctions: in Barbados these distinctions include nationality, surnames, and Caribbean identity. As a result, during the home visit, questionnaires about racial background elicit responses like "Bajan!" and "Foreparents from Guyana" and "Portuguese" and "Caribbean." These distinctions are coded according to biomedical norms as "Afro-Caribbean" in contrast to Caucasian or East Indian, which is then coded as biologically black in contrast to white or Hispanic. Race is multiple in both approaches, but biomedicine turns the valued space of contestation found in "Bajans, Africans" into the valued stability and inscribability of "25 percent Caucasian." Where vernaculars of race contain contradictions to explore multiple identities, diagnostics of race use various criteria to produce a single representation. Technological descriptors like percent of racial admixture are used in compulsive ways not reducible to their internal logics, allowing genetic admixture to be used with several other criteria as independently sufficient to diagnose race amid the moral focus in medicine of addressing health disparities. My point here is not to oppose the genetic designation of race with some reflexive contingency of identities. Rather, it is that racial and ethnic identities, like others, are used inconsistently, obsessively, and contradictorily, whether by families in household assertions or by medical researchers through genetic technologies. When these contradictory categories interact in the home visit, mutual evaluations of authority become part of the designations of race and illness that are produced.

Finding Family

The different emphases between the genetic approach and that of Bajan families were accentuated in home visit negotiations over "family." At one level, geneticists pose families as equivalent to races in the sense that both are potential sources of genetic variability: a single family can account for a gene-phenotype relationship in a population just as a race can (e.g., European genes in Pima Indians) (Barnes et al. 2001). As a family-based study, the Barbados research is valued as not open to the problems of population techniques, such as differentiation within the group (e.g., two distinct races within the population); however, the genetics team considers the complexity of families in Barbados a research conundrum.

Conflicts between genetic and Bajan emphases on family arose in interactions between the study facilitators and the participants. The genetics team must differentiate children sharing a mother but having different fathers in ways not necessary for the mother who is raising them. The researchers talked about this frequent household situation in Barbados, in conversations on the difficulties of conducting the study, and at times in print: one article written by the team explains the large number of half-sibling pairs that were included by noting "multiple partnerships are relatively common in Barbados" (Barnes et al. 1996: 42). The team and many Bajan families also emphasized differently the categorization of aunts and uncles, depending on how involved an individual had been with the rest of the family. As families decided what members to suggest to the researchers for recruitment, they made their own evaluations about kinship ties, as in this interaction between a study facilitator and an asthmatic man in his forties involved in the study, that took place during a home visit:

> FACILITATOR: You have two sisters with asthma, right?
> LESTER: Yeah, one of them, I don't think she's going to talk. But the other one will.
> FACILITATOR: Okay, can we have her number? [He gives the facilitator the phone number]
> FACILITATOR: And the other sister?
> LESTER: I don't think she will talk to you. She's not like that, she's not like that.

Lester's reluctance revealed a common decision process as participants measured helping or burdening family members. As with the meanings of asthma, negotiations over family inclusion were conducted within the genetics team, as well as between the team and the family. Team members disagreed over this—for example, whether an individual should be included in the study if his/her parents were unavailable, or whether an asthmatic man who married into an asthmatic family should be included.

The resolution of who is what kind of family member in the study facilitation is later opened to question again by the researchers. Genomic analysis of the blood samples was used to interpret the lineages to determine whether the familial relationships reported by the participants are correct. When genetic analysis reveals a reported relationship to be unlikely, a more genetically probable relationship is posited and the analysis is based on this new relationship. Further, the common genetic research practice of inferring the genotype of missing parents from the genotypes of siblings is employed. These reconstructions at times rely on racial distinctions of allele frequency as family links are adjusted according to expected relationships based on prevalence of racial gene markers (Blumenthal et al. 2003). This tinkering with kinship links forged in the home visit allowed family to be a medically negotiable object: married in or biological, inferred or self-reported, genetically probable or plausible owing to observed household relationships.

Comparing Databases

The biomedical objects I have followed here are mutually constituted in the study. Asthma measurement at times depends on ethnic categorization as, during genetic analysis, lung function estimates are adjusted for race (Huang et al. 2003). In the study comparing Barbadians and African Americans, the results found linkage to a genetic area for total IgE in the Barbadian population and for asthma in the African American population (Barnes et al. 2001). The authors noted that this linkage is dependent on the presence of another gene, and that this gene-gene-disease interaction was not found in a U.S. Caucasian and a Latin American data set. Here, meanings of gene-gene and asthma take shape in relation to each other through the particularities of research and analysis. Asthma, genes, family, and race are stabilized in their interaction.

These scientific designations are then positioned within the broader science of asthma and genetics. A database of asthmatics "of African descent" gives new racial significance to this science: the genetic research on particular ethnic populations is contrasted with biomedical asthma research that does not mention race. Asthma researchers pose prevalence, severity, and hospitalization rates among "populations of African descent" against the general population or against the findings of particular studies conducted in European countries in which the population is considered overwhelmingly white. In this process, just as divergent populations are linked as biologically black, so populations of previously unspecified race become "Caucasian."

This is the case in a study conducted by some members of the Johns Hopkins team comparing the Barbadian asthmatic participants with a population of Pennsylvania Amish. This study examined the linkage of a gene to total IgE among the Amish and to asthma among the Barbadians (Barnes et al. 1996). Here, the Bajan population (of African descent, tropical, and exposed to particular allergens) was contrasted with the Caucasian population. Through this comparison, different exposures to allergens in tropical and northern climates become part of the biologically specific racial histories.

For the genetics team, it is this specificity of race-gene-environment that differentiates their work from the strategy adopted by DeCODE, Schering-Plough, and Genome Therapeutics, in which populations are considered representative of the human genome. As discussed in chapter 3, in 2002 Schering-Plough, Genome Therapeutics, and a British university announced the association of a gene (ADAM33) with asthma. This finding has been highly influential among geneticists of asthma, and most teams have since genotyped their populations for the presence of ADAM33. Ethnic/racial distinctions are used to interpret the results, as I found in conversations with geneticists working in Puerto Rico and in the United States as part of the CSGA: the lack of a link found between ADAM33 and asthma in their population is interpreted to indicate that ADAM33 is not relevant to Hispanic or African American populations. By posing these ethnicities in contrast to Schering-Plough's population, these researchers make Schering-Plough's patient group into a Caucasian population (a different categorization than the company adopts). Genetic databases thereby become "polar with respect to each other," to use James Boon's phrasing referring to languages (1982: 133): ethnicity is used to interpret the applicability and value of databases and results, in a process of finding the lack in another's database. In this practice, databases, genes, and populations are contrasted in order to stake claims—to knowledge, to markets, to patient groups. In the process, populations are made biologically representative of ethnic groups, allowing new medical groupings of communities.

Potential in the Present

This process of database positioning reveals some of the strategic character of "race" in asthma science. As with other current biomedical research and practice, geneticists understand race to be a proxy—a tool or a model until more precise genetic, environmental, and clinical knowledge is produced that will obviate the need for these racial distinctions. The team considers these comparisons of ethnic-specific populations to be critical to finding genetic predispositions that are shared by different ethnicities. One team member described the importance to the gene-environment research of comparing the African American and Afro-Caribbean populations as black:

> If we find that the genes are the same and there are different environmental factors with the asthmatics, that would be very significant. For instance, in Baltimore we are looking at environment and genes with different endotoxins. So we might be able to find genes and specific allergic reactions. At least that's what we're shooting for.

The research is intended to locate gene-allergy interactions that are independent of race. A similar position is taken in a team article:

> Our analytic strategy for atopy consisted of two approaches, the first focused on the location of genes that could be considered as "common" across all

ethnic groups (all families were used in linkage) and the second focused on ethnic-specific effects (analysis within ethnic group). For any region providing support for linkage in the total family collection, that region can then be decomposed into the contribution from each ethnic group. In this manner, a relatively equal contribution would suggest a common gene in a common pathway that could increase genetic risk of atopy, while failure of an ethnic group to support linkage could suggest that the evidence was dependent upon the founding population allele frequency or an interaction of the specific locus with a specific allergen (or environmental factor). (Blumenthal et al. 2003: 8)

Ethnic difference is identified with family, or geographic area, as a contributing factor that must be contrasted in order to find objects that transcend the contrast. Race in this genetic biomedicine is simultaneously a biology (because it is genetic), an approximation (because it is based on self-identification), and a strategy (because it is a temporary step on the path to more precise characterization of diseases and medication response).

This interpretation of race as a proxy emphasizes an idealized future, as focus is placed on the coming medicine that will be created by the speed and scale of genomic technologies and research. Here, genetic research as cumulative is critical to its significance: each genetic, gene-gene, or gene-environment study is considered to contribute to knowledge about the interaction of gene, environment, and population. In this process, genomic databases and collaborative efforts can combine analyses, making statistically nonsignificant results potentially significant. For example, comparison of the Barbadian and Amish populations suggested an association of asthma with a chromosomal region—an association not considered significantly strong when the populations were analyzed independently. Biomedical research on race-disease links is premised on ideals of cumulative potential.

This is not restricted to the genetic aspect of the research: one of the researchers involved in the environmental aspect of the gene-environment studies explained that the filters put into homes collect data on many different possible allergens, but during analysis some must be selected to the exclusion of others. As a result, the researchers have decided to wait to analyze filters that have been used in the studies: "Each analysis destroys a filter, so we will wait until we know what to test for, until the science catches up. So we've decided to keep them until then." The practice of waiting for the science to catch up is increasing in biomedical research based on technologies that can process enormous amounts of data: this focus on the future is generative of practices in the present that are shaping meanings of gene-environment-race-disease.

The Asthmatic's Genes

Race is the basis for the significance of the asthma study to the science of disease genetics; the research is conducted on Barbadians insofar as they are considered representative of African Americans. The Bajan families, by contrast, never talked about race in discussing why they entered the study or the causes of asthma. As discussed in chapter 6, the Bajan families partially value the genetics teams as associated with the expertise, technology, and money of U.S. medicine; this is also what makes the study strange to them. The purpose of the study, the blood tubes and needles, and the technologies were all treated as foreign and laden in the home visit encounters. When parents questioned the researchers about the study and its purpose, at times the arcane aspect of the gene was maintained, and DNA and the use of the blood remained vague and associated with the technologies and biomedical perspective of the team. At other times, mothers and fathers would continue to question, in an attempt to give shape to the nebulous meanings of the technologies and expertise of genetic research. In these interactions, researchers and facilitators would link genes to blood and family history as involved in the presence and severity of asthma. This presentation largely echoed the consent form, which included the common posing of family history and genes:

> Why is this research being done?
> This research is being done to try and find genes that cause asthma and allergies. We know that asthma/allergies are often found in several members of the same family. Why is this? One idea is that the tendency to asthma is passed down from one or both parents to the child (it is inherited).

(The form went on to discuss environmental causes of asthma and allergies.) These explanations led many participants to speculate on the familial character of asthma; as one mother remarked, "Then it must come from her father's side." These genetic genealogies were used to reinterpret family narratives about health, as I argued in chapter 6.

As "genes" inscribe family stories into a linear descent of illness, the technologies gave their role an aura of authoritative specificity. The spirometer and computer by which lung function is measured provided a highly visible and direct indication of asthma for the participants. They associated the technology with more exact measurements of their illness than those considered available to other health practitioners.[8] At the same time, this specificity remained opaque and arcane.

For many families, the foreign and unknown aspects of the research included a level of danger. The amount of blood being drawn and the use of the blood were almost invariably a source of apprehension for the families. In almost every home visit, these worries were the catalyst to ask about the purpose of the research. In response to the fears about the amount of blood being drawn, the study facilitators would indicate how small the amount was in comparison to the amount of blood in the body. Some participants asked further questions about the meaning of genes. In one case, a teenage boy fainted for several seconds during the drawing of blood. His mother became very worried and wanted to know how much blood had been taken, and whether this was the same amount as had been taken from others. The mother then turned her attention to the purpose of the study, asking rapidly what the blood was needed for, what genes are, and whether the research would help asthmatics. Her continued participation in this process reveals the level of value she (like others) placed on some kind of personalized attention to, particularly, her children's illness.

As discussed in chapter 6, the families contrasted this attention with their experience in the public health care system. The genetics team talked about this motive. I had the following interaction with one study facilitator early in my fieldwork:

FACILITATOR: People are very willing to help, to be part of the study. In the…study I'm working on, they're not being paid, and people are willing to be part of it.

AUTHOR: Is that because people are happy with the care here?

FACILITATOR: It's because people are *not* happy with the care here.…They can't handle the demand. If you go into the Hospital at ten at night, you will get out at six the next morning.

This facilitator mentioned participants expressing their frustration with the care they had received for their asthma, or more often their children's asthma. I saw several such moments in home visits. One mother believed that her daughter had become asthmatic due to a reaction to a pain medication she had received at the hospital. Another talked about her eleven-year-old daughter having to go to the hospital for her asthma directly after returning from the polyclinic. In these interactions, mothers gave voice to their anger and fears; there was little requested from the team except to acknowledge these problems. These mothers turn the researchers into witnesses to their hardships: the personalized attention of the study was partially this acknowledgment of the mothers' difficulties within the Barbadian medical system.

Occasionally, however, the families desired more medical action from the genetics team, usually in the form of specific information. During one home visit, an elderly woman got out a box of medicines and asked a genetics team member to explain the purpose of the various medications she had been prescribed, for asthma and otherwise. In another home visit, a mother of two asthmatics asked a geneticist why her current (reliever) inhaler (Berotec) seemed different from her previously prescribed (reliever) inhaler (Ventolin). Since Berotec is not available in the United States, the geneticist was unfamiliar with the inhaler but after some discussion with other team members, explained to the woman that this was a reliever inhaler, different from the preventive inhalers. The mother asked what the side effects were. The geneticist responded with "nervousness" and "makes your heart race." The genetics team thus provides redress to the secretive and dangerous silence about medications found in the doctor's office, in the views of the patients. But, as indicated in chapter 6, this search for medical answers from foreign expertise includes skepticism about what is found. The families I talked with maintain a conflicted perspective of the research as personalized attention with little practical use. This extended to their use of the study results.

Translating Test Results

The complex mix of skepticism, hope, and belief was particularly visible in how the participants used the allergen test results. This standardized test involves pricking the skin to assess reactivity to various allergens, including types of mold, cockroaches, grasses, dog and cat dander, and pollen from trees. Participant families receive a list of allergens to which each family member reacts. These are the only individualized results given to the participants; during the home visit many asked about the genetic results, but the study policy is that DNA results are not given to participants.[9]

Almost all of the families talked about these allergen test results when discussing the value of the research with me. Celia Hunt explained, "They sent back a whole listing of things to me, so now I know what I am allergic to, what each child is allergic to, their father. And I was able then to give my personal doctor part of the document so that he can go along that line with us." One of Celia's sons had serious asthma attacks often and at unknown times, and was continuing to not take his inhaled steroid. When I asked what had resulted from giving the doctor the allergen test results, Celia said that nothing had really changed. I asked whether she had made any changes based on her participation in the genetics study, and she told me she had not. This is not surprising given the nature of the allergen results, which are difficult to act on. What is significant is that this pattern was true for all of the participants who mentioned the value of the allergen tests: all expressed appreciation about knowing the triggers, and none had changed their behavior because of it. When I asked one mother what she thought about the sheet with the allergen test results, she remarked, "What I think about it? It help." She then paused for a long time, and added, · "I think...you know, I don't understand it." Another mother told me about what she had gained from the study: "They took blood and then they had this—like the grass and the roach and the different things to test what they are allergic to." I asked her if she had done anything with this list. She responded, "Well. Roach, I really—in some cases the roach running, and we already sterilize to a point. Grass—they don't be in grass. Cats, and rats, and dogs, but I ain't got no cats or dogs in here."

The value of the allergen test in these discussions was not as a plan for action; instead, the results comprised biomedical attention to the vagaries of asthma experience and medical care. For some, like Frank Lawrence, the study results were valued as helpful for other asthmatics:

> Personally, I don't think it [the genetics study] make no difference. It didn't make no difference to me, right, because we had he [his son] under control already, right, because we never really take chances after we find out he an asthmatic, right? But and the allergy test and things only tell you really what you're allergic to. So, but the test itself, I feel, you get some good information that could work with other asthmatics. But me personally, it didn't really make no difference.

For Frank and some other participants, the allergen test results and the study were of no direct use, only more abstractly possibly useful to others. One asthmatic in her twenties viewed the allergen test as helping make sense of the frightening uncertainty of when and why an attack would happen: the test gave shape to asthma by listing causes that might occur at specific times. And she felt involvement in the study separated her from other asthmatics who were still caught in the instability of not having such a list.

Cathy Boxer focused not on the results but on the allergen test itself:

> You now realize that there are tests out there to find out if your lungs are
> damaged, what you're allergic to, and you find out because of the study, you
> know, it is nothing that is generally done. But of course I know that you can
> do it in Barbados if you do pay. That there are ways to get these things done,
> but it just open your eyes that there are tests and there are diagnoses and
> ways to find out, you know, about your asthma, about the damage done to
> your lungs. So it was surprising to know that those things exist. But the aver-
> age asthmatic doesn't know that it exists.

For Cathy, these tests were an aid in understanding the experience of
asthma, similar to the consumption of medicines and pharmaceutical
company leaflets: they provide tangible means of understanding the arcane
of technological, medical, and scientific practice. Significantly, such consumption is restricted, in her account, to those who can pay.[10] The value
of the genetic research is generated by the context of a Barbadian asthma
community, the "average asthmatic," who must live with the instability of
the lack of diagnostics.

Cathy's sister Diane, who also had not changed her behavior as a result
of the study, talked about the importance of the allergen test. She contrasted
her having the list with the experience of other asthmatics:

> Honestly some people do have attacks and you can ask them, "Okay, what
> did you do to get this?" Or, "Were you around something that caused?"—
> Some people honestly get attacks through trial and error. And if they are vig-
> ilant with themselves, they might remember, "Okay, I was around a chemical
> yesterday, that is what caused that." Or "I smelled somebody's perfume, or
> something." But apart from that, some people don't know what cause the
> attacks.

As Diane continued to talk, I had a vague sense that she was talking about
herself—that she was included in this group of asthmatics who have to live
with the uncertainty of not knowing the causes that bring on an attack. In
any case, the allergen test results for Diane were an idealized (not realized)
intervention on this uncertainty: they have value not as the basis for action
on the precarious asthmatic experience, but as a symbolic reduction of this
precariousness.

In these accounts, the test results were a concrete object that was personalized. Being specific, the list brought the genetics study and therefore

biomedical knowledge into the domestic space where it could be manipulated and used. But this concreteness is paradoxically based on maintaining
its arcane, unknown character. The results are only useful insofar as they
are symbolic; they lack practical significance (e.g., "ain't got no dogs or cats
here"). They were valued in that they keep an association with unknown
expertise.[11] This then is not a simple translation of the arcane into the familiar, of the abstract into the practical: part of the fundamental foreign-
ness of scientific and biomedical practices is maintained in the translation
into the asthmatic experience, allowing it to have a symbolic potential.

The allergen tests then, like the oral steroids, are anomalies. They are associated by the families with U.S.-based expertise, valued as non-Barbadian
medical care that separates the family from the regular Bajan asthmatic,
and they are simultaneously made Bajan, domestic. They are used at once
to criticize Barbadian medical care, make the strangeness of the genetics
research knowable, and maintain this unknowability of scientific expertise
as having value.

The Biomedical Domestic Space

In a collaborative gene-environment study being conducted by the Johns
Hopkins genetics group that was beginning during my fieldwork, researchers place three metallic cylinders in the asthmatic's home. These cylinders
remain in the home for weeks, measuring tobacco and other types of smoke,
air pollution, dust, and other particles. The team thereby brings domestic environmental analyses that are not available in the government intervention
on asthma. During a home visit for this study, a man asked what the purpose
of the study was, as the team looked for an electrical outlet. One researcher
responded to look at the environment and pollution. The man asked, "Is
asthma hereditary?" The researcher responded that it was. The man continued, "So, this is really studying lifestyle." The researcher responded that this
was studying what was both outside and inside the home, not restricted
to the man's behavior. In these exchanges, heredity and environment are
made newly significant for families. The participants use this intrusion: allowing the researchers, blood tubes and needles, computers, and spirometers into their homes invites a reshaping of their domestic space. The parent is thereby intervening in the frightening unknown of his or her child's
illness, the frustration with the extant system, and linking the family with
the expertise and funding of the United States. The study becomes a kind of
medical care, in their view. The domestic space becomes a site of knowledge
production and of action around their children's disease. Their multiple

evaluations of the source and techniques of the researchers—as medical, as American, as "experts"—is integrated into the meanings they make of asthma causes like "lifestyle," "genetic," and "allergic."

Conclusion: Foundational Absences

The contrasting emphases of the home visit accentuate the ways international biomedical research is foundationally hybrid (a thorny concept in current social criticism[12]). The way that disease, gene, and race are used is structural: the terms are inherently contradictory. This applies to the gamut of signification that I have explored here: asthma as wheeze and medication response, as genetic and self-identified; race as Afro-Caribbean not European, as Barbadian not Guyanese, as strategic but ontological, also genetic and self-identified; genetic research as medical intervention, as potential, as symbol of international markets, of American expertise and money, as future amid present practice. The participants have views of asthma, ethnicity, family, and patienthood that are contrastive to the study, at times intentionally. Through these contradictions these terms can have multiple meanings, and therefore myriad effect giving them, as all myths, their facility. But their use is not free play: this is not social construction, but instead operations (always) within systems of meaning. This contingency and stability, peculiar to myths since Lévi-Strauss's work, is the sense in which race-gene-disease is being forged relationally while moving medicine in particular directions.

The generic human genome, as everyone's and no one's, only has meaning in relation to the deviations from it: the genetic disease, the predisposition, the ethnic, geographic, or otherwise other population. It is these deviations that DeCODE, Schering-Plough, and the Collaborative Study on Genetics of Asthma are searching for in making a patient group representative of a population. Doing so positions databases in terms of medical utility, intervention, and markets. Race-disease links are effected in this process. The framing of the analytic use of race as a tool, a proxy, a "place holder," on the path to more particular, exact, individualized, or informative biological markers engenders research and medical practices. This tool is shifting race by linking divergent populations through particular research projects on diseases and pharmaceuticals. "Environment" takes shape as chemicals, dust, roadwork, and livestock ownership are turned into levels of IgE and particulate matter in interaction with genetic predispositions. Asthma severity is turned into use of pharmaceuticals and facilities alongside wheezing. Government officials take up these translations into

a biology of race and disease. These biomedical logics link asthma diagnosis with pharmaceuticals; health intervention with adherence discourse;
and health disparities with genetic research.

George Steiner gives us a characteristically eloquent critique of language
use as information flow:

> Thus it is inaccurate and theoretically spurious to schematize language as
> "information" or to identify language, be it unspoken or vocalized, with
> "communication." The latter term will serve only if it includes, if it places
> emphasis on, what is *not* said in the saying, what is said only partially, al-
> lusively or with intent to screen. Human speech conceals far more than it
> confides; it blurs much more than it defines; it distances more than it con-
> nects. (1998: 240)

When we include science as a language, the passage draws attention to
what is lacking in the metaphor of the building of knowledge creating
an increasingly complete structure. We must attend to the ways scientific
approaches, like all others, conceal as they confide. Steiner's wording emphasizes not only the constitutive absences in language but also its enacted
aspect, the significance of intent, of relationships between speaker and listener. This sociality is foundational to the ways race and disease are being
recast in the internationalization of biomedicine. In exchanges between
families, researchers, and facilitators, evaluations of the giver and receiver
are constitutive. Expertise is diversely assessed, for example, as market-
driven—useful as bringing funded research or denigrated as biased—and as
multinational—inapplicable to Barbadian specificities or free of Barbadian
troubles. These evaluations introduce fundamental contradictions in the
extension of pharmaceuticalization and biomedicalization.

Families exhibit such contradictions in their interpretation and use of
the genetic research. They experience and evaluate a moral responsibility
of the mother as caregiver, a focus on pharmaceutical adherence as public
health, and the family as basis of asthma genetics. They engage these discourses inconsistently, at times identifying with, elsewhere angrily criticiz-
ing, their potency in medical care and knowledge. Patient consumption of
oral steroids—hoarded rather than taken as prescribed—is a commentary
on medicine in Barbados. Similarly, participation in the research is a rejection of a biomedicalized Barbadian government medical care. This results
in ambivalent interpretations of the study results: the allergen test is seen
on one hand as individualized, my son's, a solidarity with the research, and
simultaneously as foreign, strange, arcane, useless. Similarly, the doctors'

categorization of asthma is skeptically consumed: made ironic, at times laughed at in its narrow focus, it is also employed and searched out. These families use the discourses they ridicule, enact identities made from discourses they provisionally reject. This signification differs with one precluding falsehood, contradiction, and ambiguities: the stability of medical categories can be undone with humor without losing salience.

This excess of the home visit exchange warns against consistent representations of medical categories. The interactions between scientists and Bajans reveal that medical categories and objects are used compulsively, strangely, unpredictably—for example, in percentage of Caucasian admixture, Caribbean as a biology, or allergen tests as personal attention with no utility. This plurality is often lost in scientific—and anthropological—depictions. Such representations tend to preclude the possibility of overlap, of vagueness, of contradictory placement. The genetic discourse of race is peculiar not because it claims to be authoritative (what does not?) but because it claims to be consistent, to have a single criterion universally applicable. Unequivocal and objectified means of identification are common: vernaculars of race claim just as much certainty, truth, and authority as do genetic ones. But vernaculars tend to allow a (valued) space for multiplicity and inconsistency. This is what lets "Bajans, Africans" to continue to be held alongside "Bajan" as competing, not clearly demarcated, but nonetheless strongly held and unequivocal concepts of racial identity. Scientific and medical representations erase the multiplicity and inconsistencies of race that occur as researchers and medical practitioners interact with patients and families. But this is not necessarily unique to genetics—such hyperconsistency is also found in cultural anthropologists' and sociologists' claims to have an unproblematic answer to the quandary of race.

The plurality of inconsistent reflections and interpretations among the families suggests a space for valued multiplicity that gives pause to our biomedical and anthropological certainties, as we diagnose race, disease, and biomedicalization.

Chapter 9

Biomedical and
Anthropological Excesses

Unlikely Genetics

In the extensive conversations I had with families about dust, the category
had a particularly vague valence. Early in my fieldwork, I continually tried
to reduce this ambiguity by asking people to tell me the one or several com-
ponents that make up this dust. I failed, and only belatedly came to real-
ize that this vagueness was integral to the concept. Asthma specialists and
researchers in Barbados offered several competing definitions: the sands
and allergens brought from the Sahara by the winds; the exhaust from the
increased automobile use; the airborne debris produced by roadwork; finally, there was brief mention made of the soil being dustier as a result of
erosion and damage caused by the economic reliance on sugar cane. However, among Barbadians not involved in medicine or research that I spoke
with, the ambiguity of dust was not due to varying definitions, but rather
a fundamental slippage in the category. Such vagueness made the category
usable for multiple criticisms. Cathy and Diane Boxer discussed the causes
of asthma in Barbados with their mother:

> CATHY: I think it is the air too! Because how can—[indicating her mother]
> you are an adult! Like my mother now, you started wheezing now, how?
> MOTHER: A couple of years ago.

CATHY: A couple of years ago, in your forties, right?

MOTHER: I was like in my late thirties, in my thirties, the dust.

CATHY: Exactly, right, and that never used to affect her before.

MOTHER: Right.

CATHY: To me it's more than just—

MOTHER: It's the dust and smoke—

CATHY: It's the atmosphere, man, the atmosphere is dirty—.

DIANE: It's the atmosphere change, a definite atmosphere change.

MOTHER: I feel it is more chemicals and the carbon monoxide.

CATHY: Exactly. The air is just not clean. You know, sometimes you can actually feel yourself catching an asthma attack just being outside in the open! You can smell things that make you feel yourself short of breath.

MOTHER: You don't have to exert yourself.

This integral vagueness is what allows dust to be a source of boundaries between pollution and purity (see Douglas 1966) in changes wrought by modernization, industrialization, and community practices.

My claim is that this contradictory character is also found in the medical objects I have explored here. Race in current biomedicine has a basic ambiguity that allows the category to operate differently in different contexts. The urgency of research on race and disease, the moral and market pressure to address disparities and minority populations, results in a kind of expedient pragmatic approach to race in biomedicine: multiple criteria are considered independently sufficient for categorization. Self-identification, inferring ancestry, parental identification, country of origin, and current geographic location are each used as diagnostic of race, at times interchangeably. Asthma in biomedicine is similarly variably defined: it is diagnosable by the patient's response to medication or to allergens, or by the patient's history, with severity measured by the number of emergency room visits, the amount of medication used, or the patient's perspective. But where the vagueness of dust can be valued and accentuated in vernaculars, such contradictions are devalued and thereby often hidden in official discourses, like biomedicine and anthropology.

This implied consistency that masks contradictions is found when biomedical technologies are used to provide specific measurements of variable objects, in what I have called "hyperdiagnostics." Asthma is measured in numbers of eosinophils, total serum IgE levels, percentage of lung response to methacholine; the search for gene-race-disease links gives us numbers like the percentage of Caucasians with slow metabolizing gene variants. And these hyperdiagnoses reinforce each other, allowing ethnic correction of lung response during spirometry, and correlation of asthma-associated genetic variants with percentage of African ancestry.

Such diagnostics increasingly rely on divergent populations. With the focus on genomics, institutions like the FDA, NIH, and pharmaceutical companies are drawing biological links between disease populations. The pressure to address minorities, to find therapeutic markets, and to target and explain disparities, along with the increasing difficulty of conducting medical research on U.S. populations, results in expanded efforts to make biological links between populations in the United States and Western Europe with poorer countries. These projects often rely on local governments for access to patients, facilitation of research, and robust medical records.

Biomedical partnerships are thereby forged between governments and multinational companies and British and U.S. medical institutions. These partnerships rely on a "genetic futurism": an evaluation of genetics as the medicine of tomorrow, with the attendant value of being at the forefront of the global medical interventions. The governments portray their nations as biomedical markets to attract such research—in the case of Barbados, as biologically black disease populations. In so doing, the Barbadian government draws on values of nationalism (contrasting the medical sophistication of Barbados with other Caribbean countries) and internationalism (taking part in the course of biomedical progress). The moral and social necessity of intervention is interpolated into genetics of race and disease: the nation poses its population as black and genetically relevant in order to gain from the biomedical discoveries to come; the genetics team poses the participants as black in constituting a database on those with the greater burden of disease; and the pharmaceutical industry poses them as black in need of intervention on their lack of adherence to treatment. Similarly, once ethnically specific genetic predispositions or medications are located, their use along racial lines is morally required. The proposed genetic propensity of black people toward severe asthma has significance in a system of meanings as patients, as nonadherent, as research subjects, as excessively suffering from disease. The space of race and disease is thereby knowable through the study of genome-environment.

As a result, a nexus of biology-disease-race is constituted as a target for interventions. Barbadian asthmatics become a black database, which morally needs to be analyzed so that the market or state can intervene. The biomedical research attending to the biology of the race becomes a kind of state care, as health disparities are linked to genes. Race in Barbados can be exchanged with race in the United States, just as Bajan meanings of asthma can be substituted for biomedical meanings through questionnaires in order to medically intervene on minority groups.

This contextual use and meaning link the production and consumption of biomedicine in subtle ways. Medical practitioners make use of the genetics research they come across in interactions at conferences and medical practice. This operates by involution as various otherwise unrelated diseases are linked through genetic research on a particular population. Such involution is facilitated by the health care system. (As a result, in countries like Iceland and Barbados, the contingency of how diseases are categorized in public health programs becomes part of the significance of the genetics database.) Statements on admixture give new genetic meanings to racial histories. Through these practices, the creation and use of biomedical knowledge are newly soldered, as countries incorporate genetic research in unlikely ways.

Medicine is consequently reconfigured. Through a national formulary, the state forges a public health intervention that requires constant adjustment to international pharmaceutical markets. Postcolonial states utilize what they consider to be problematic biomedical practices (market-driven research, pharmaceutical pamphlets as education) to meet medical needs. The plurality of asthma combines with a pressure to unambiguously diagnose the condition to create an expansive category, independently diagnosable through medication response, presence of wheeze, or family history. Conditions like cancer, diabetes, and obesity become associated with biological race. These practices create new categories: the potential asthmatic—genetically predisposed, diagnosed with asthma without ever having had an attack; the pharmaceutical citizen—a patient-consumer responsible for proper adherence; glaucoma as a black person's disease; a genetically black mother participant—medicalized as caretaker of the asthmatic. Such discursive objects are used as parents make decisions about their children's health, as doctors decide on kinds of treatment, and as government officials make public policy.

Categorical Ambiguities

But these practices are implemented with a foundational critique that makes them unstable. The marketization of public health is a kind of frustrated globalism: a postcolonial government's particular combination of anger and pride at multinational influence on the state. The pharmaceutical is valued as a resource-poor intervention—an expedient fix more tenable than structural changes—but its role in public health in Barbados is criticized by the Drug Service committee members who make it central to policy. Physicians advertise pharmaceuticals in their offices while bitterly reflecting on this runaway commerce-based state medicine. And study facilitators simultaneously value and disbelieve the potential applicability of the research to Barbados. This mix of hope and skepticism, participation and criticism, of critique and want, is constitutive of the efficacy of international biomedical practices in the postcolonial country.

Such contradictions both facilitate biomedical categorization and are the source of alternatives to them. If race had no more meaning than the presence of a set of genetic markers, it would have little utility and less currency among medical practitioners or families. Its "proxy" nature—that appearance can stand for genetics, or self-identity for disease propensity—is not incidental but foundational. If pharmaceuticalization was simply pharmaceutical companies determining public health techniques, government representatives in countries like Barbados would not enact it: in order to be accepted, industry agendas have to be posed as refusable by autonomous governments. The play of rejection and acceptance is fundamental to implementation, as reflection on categories is integral to their use. The genetic research is considered authoritative and absurd by medical practitioners, changing medical techniques even as its utility is rejected. The social medicine pharmaceutical is a discursive object only possible amid its own undermining: the denouncing of the excesses and narrow focus of global markets. The medicalized mother as a category fraught with power would have little cache among families if it was not also a source of pride and strength for women.[1] The genetically black asthmatic is thus created in foundationally contested spaces that nonetheless have an effect on care, families, and nations.

A basic instability is introduced by these moments of use and ridicule, how we make sense of what we reject, how we employ what we undermine. In these ambivalent moments, mutually inconsistent meanings not only can be maintained but also can reinforce each other.[2] Among government officials, frustration with the influence of the pharmaceutical industry can heighten the simultaneous pride in gaining from this influence. Among the participant families, the vague significance of the allergen test can be the source of its concrete utility. Such reflection makes the uses of discourses difficult to interpret. Pharmaceuticalization is a process of postcolonial governments utilizing the pharmaceutical as a social good, and yet in the moments of ambivalence and reversals that comprise this process, it is already one step removed from this interpretation called "pharmaceuticalization." Similarly genetic futurism: medical practitioners come to see asthma and race as genetically linked, a bond only knowable through so-phisticated and opaque technologies and expertise, and yet in this proc-ess they come to denounce the relevance and necessity of such technology and expertise, opening alternatives even as they implement this "genetic futurism." Hierarchies in expertise and moral logics not only are often re-versed they are at heart reversible[3] (e.g., doctor diagnostics versus family knowledge, American geneticist biomedicine versus Barbadian physician experience, and pharmaceutical company as benefactor versus Formulary Committee as beneficiary). This reversibility is what makes analysis of power/knowledge a thorny, contradictory (and rich) practice.

These schismogenics of cultural meanings suggest oscillations that are foundational to biomedical objects and are too often erased in our diag-noses of disease, markets, and medicine.[4] This cultural movement includes the excesses of biomedical creation and use: the hoarding of unused medi-cines; the plethora of side effects imagined within the strange lack of such in the doctor's office; the extraordinary specificity of measurements of race and of asthma, a kind of obsessive use of precision; the pharmaceutical as social and preventive medicine; gene, race, and asthma as categories that go haywire in their formation and interpretation. Such cultural use produces strange objects like the potential asthmatic, 25 percent Caucasian Barbadi-ans, 80 percent asthma prevalence, the morally and medically nonadherent mother, and inhaled steroids that have none of the side effects of steroids. These objects are created by mutual exaggerations in the exchanges that comprise science and medicine.

To emphasize the way these excesses place our diagnoses of power, ex-pertise, and political economy into doubt, I have looked to anthropological tools that can be productively applied to themselves (e.g., Bateson's schis-mogenesis, Mauss's exchange, Levi-Strauss's myths, Geertz's winks (on all of these, see Boon 1999)). Bateson's schismogenesis, like Mauss's exchange, and Lévi-Strauss's structuralism, offers a critique of any model of maxi-mization, including of analytic approaches. As Boon (1999) has shown: in Mauss's exchange, mutual extremes always involve excess and dearth, un-deremphasized in Marx's (or any other) utilitarian model; Lévi-Strauss's myths, only having significance and existing by contrast, only allow a science-by-contrast, a mythology-as-myth-making that while motivated from within, is arbitrary from without; and Bateson's schismogenics make attempts at maximization into either complementary or symmetrical re-lations of pathological reliance. These tools offer analyses that avoid the distancing of diagnosis, in which recognition of a social, cultural, or psy-chological malady seems to inoculate the diagnoser. The multivalence of discourses warns against any radical consistency that would allow the various depictions offered by different anthropologists to be stacked up without slippage in the building of an edifice representing globalization, modernity, biomedicine, science, subjectivity.

In this portrayal I have tried to attend to my own ambivalence—my criticisms of neoliberal practices, the pharmaceutical industry, and biomedical categorization, and my conviction that such critiques tend to enact what they attempt to undermine: the analytic categorization that precludes listening for further subtleties, that ends dialogue. In writing of contradiction, I have struggled to remain contradictory. My own approach to this quandary has been to try to portray my interpretations, like the "pharmaceutical citizen" and "geneticization" of asthma and race, while also portraying how these interpretations unravel or fail because these practices integrate critical reflection on them. By following the ways families, practitioners, geneticists, and officials exceed our analytic conclusions, I try to use them as broken interpretations.[5] I meant to explore what a science or anthropology might look like that acknowledges a space for analytic tools as multiple and vague as the Bajan notion of dust. Given the prevalence of such objects—"asthma" in American medicine, "race" in bioscience, "science" in anthropology—some integrated acceptance of such might be salutary: a space for contradiction, for valued vagueness, might open new interpretations of the global, familial, and corporate systems that we analyze and take part in.

The translation of the populations and practices I have explored here into the science of genetics generates particular meanings of disease, race, and genes that form the trajectory of biomedicine. Opposing meanings are foundational: race as strategic but ontological, "African, Bajan"; Barbados as biomedical leader and as at the mercy of biomedical practice; and genetics as a precise practice necessary to understanding race-disease and as a vague object. By attending to contradiction, we can see moments in which biomedical, or economic, or social categories are placed into quotes, where their limits are examined, played with, and criticized in ways that are constitutive of their import. We can attend to how such modern objects are read, translated, created, employed, and consumed, with excess and with reflexivity that escape our analytic reach.

Notes

Introduction: Vernaculars in Race and Disease Science

1. Pharmaceutical industry interest is based on the idea that defining the genetic basis for disease can lead to targets for new medications and that pharmacogenomics is expected to reduce adverse drug reactions and allow drugs that would otherwise be rejected as unsafe to reach the market. This focus occurs within the context of diminishing discoveries of new types of medications (new molecular entities) since the 1960s, resulting in increased attention on finding markets for existing pharmaceuticals (see Angell 2004; Goozner 2004). This level of attention and interest has resulted in projects studying genetic predispositions for various diseases, including cancer, heart disease, and respiratory conditions, and the genetics of medication response to, for example, antihypertensives, chemotherapeutics, antidepressants, and antiepileptics.

2. In medical journals, the focus has been on the possible reduction in adverse drug reactions, the current impact of which is cited in either economic terms (cost to health care) or mortality rates (an often-cited study found that such reactions are the fourth to sixth leading cause of death in the United States, which Adam Hedgecoe (2004) notes has become a kind of mantra in pharmacogenomics). Reduction in the cost and risk of clinical trials is also frequently noted as a possible benefit of pharmacogenomic research.

3. Such discussion is accompanied by a literature on the potential ethical, legal, and social issues from bioethicists, legal experts, historians, and medical professionals (see e.g., Anderlik and Rothstein 2001; Reilly 2001; Rothstein and Epps 2001; Califano et al. 2002; Issa 2002; Rothstein 2003). Legal experts have examined possible issues of health insurance discrimination and pharmaceutical industry targeting based on the categorization of some individuals as less cost-effective to treat (Rothstein and Epps 2001).

Medical practitioners, bioethicists, and legal experts have examined informed consent and privacy issues, including the potential impact for communities with a pharmacogenomic predisposition (Anderlik and Rothstein 2001; Issa 2002). The National Institutes of Health (NIH) has created a pharmacogenetics advisory group to explore these issues. This group examines the impact that genetic-based medicine might have on particular populations, focusing on issues of informed consent and authorizing individuals to represent communities.

4. The forms that these changes are taking have received considerable anthropological attention in the last ten years. These accounts have explored the cultural valence of genetic discourse (Nelkin and Lindee 1995; Haraway 1997); configurations of economic, political, legal, social, and technical trajectories by which genomics is produced (Pálsson and Rabinow 1999; Rabinow 1999); the categorizations of populations through genetic databases and community involvement (Rabinow 1992; Foster and Sharp 2002; Lock 2002); and patient uses of genetic technology and research (Rapp 1999, 2000, and 2003; Taussig et al. 2003) (see Fischer 2001 for a discussion linking such anthropological work on genetics to broader biomedical assemblages of ethics, institutions, techniques, and affect). These analyses have revealed the interlinking roles of institutions, patient families, and markets in the production and impact of genomic research.

5. In Barbados there is a politics to using the more formal term "Barbadian" instead of the more "vernacular" "Bajan." Since my informants varied in their approaches to this politics, I adopt Carla Freeman's approach (2000) of using both interchangeably.

6. For examples of such a focus in biomedical clinical trials, see Epstein 1996; Lowy 2000; Good 2001).

7. As Dell Hymes painstakingly demonstrates using myths from the Chinook (1977), the same myths can have divergent meanings for different groups in a culture, as they take on meaning contrastively, and contradiction and contestation are central to the performance of meaning.

8. See Annemarie Mol's work (1998) for a subtle exploration of disease as performed. In her account, there are multiple atheroscleroses at work in a Dutch hospital. She traces the variation in techniques by which atherosclerosis is approached and acted on, in her interest in shifting the analytic focus from representation to performance.

9. On culture as multiple, contested, ironic, see Geertz 1973; Boon 1982 and 1999; and Handler and Segal 1999.

10. Claude Lévi-Strauss writes (1983: 183), "For, in the 'upside down' world that was the state of nature before the birth of civilization, all future things had to have their counterpart, even if only in a negative form, which was a kind of guarantee of their future existence. The opossum being…the reverse pattern of absent agriculture, was an indication of what its future form would be, and at the same time,…it is the instrument whereby men obtain agriculture. The introduction of agriculture by the opossum is therefore the result of the transformation of a mode of being into its converse. A logical opposition is projected in time in the form of a relation of cause and effect. What creature could be better suited than the opossum to reconcile the two functions? Its marsupial nature combines antithetical characteristics, which become complementary only in it. For the opossums is the best of wetnurses, and yet it stinks."

11. Bulmer is also particularly attentive to the ways ideas, sentiments, and perspectives are not easily stabilized for analysis, given as they are to relational differentiation.

He consistently hints at the ways narratives and categorizations subtly respond to the interaction between speaker and listener: "In elucidating the principles which underlie Karam taxonomy at this level one of the problems is that Karam appear to take a great deal of this very much for granted, in much the same way that one takes the grammar or the phonology of one's mother-tongue for granted. It is only where distinctions are patently rather difficult to maintain, as where morphologically extremely similar small furred animals are divided among three different taxa, or where they know some other people classify creatures differently, as with cassowaries and birds, that they have ready-made explanations" (1970: 169). "There are probably other features which Karam could point to if they were pressed for additional information" (176). Bulmer's reflections see meaning-making as in motion.

Chapter 1. Contestations of Race

1. The uses of genetics of race are not limited to medicine: for example, companies offer profiling of suspects for law-enforcement agencies and in legal cases and identification of racial ancestry for individual consumers.

2. Keith Wailoo (1997) shows that this one-to-one association was also used to promote segregation and limit immigration through the 1920s, 1930s, and 1940s. He argues that technology was intricately linked to this association through the use of the diagnostic, Emmel's test, which did not distinguish people with sickle cell anemia from heterozygotes for the sickle cell trait. The technology-disease link was used in making the test a means of determining black ancestry.

3. In his lectures (2003), Michel Foucault traces modern meanings of race to the narrative histories of the peoples of Europe; race emerged as a counter-history in opposition to the discourse of the people as one with the Sovereign. In his analysis, this discourse of race split into class and biologico-medical discourses, the latter of which became the modern meanings and deployments of race. For an extended discussion of Foucault's argument, see Stoler 1995.

4. More recent analyses have focused particularly on the colonies, emphasizing the contextual, variable, and heterogeneous ways that race was deployed and shaped in colonial encounters. Ann Stoler (1995) draws on and critiques Foucault's lectures on race in her study of racial meanings in colonial contexts. She argues that concepts of purity; the goal of civilizing; and racial attributes of sexuality and desire were all constituted in colonial practices. Waltraud Ernst (1999a) focuses on the variability of race in psychiatric institutions in the colonies. Gyan Prakash (1999) shows the interaction of religious, physical, and social characterizations in forming the contextual meaning of peoples in colonial India. Homi Bhabha (1994) argues that this contingency in the colonial experience of meanings of modernity was constitutive of European identity. Bhabha thereby directs attention to the contradictory in conceptualizations of modernity, including ideas of race. This contradiction is the space of prior ideals, alternative values, the readily apparent gaps between descriptions of modernity and the colonial experience.

5. Analyses of race in the colonies reveal the centrality of medicine and disease to the constitution of racial meanings. Historians have shown that communicable diseases were used to shape approaches to race in the colonies. David Arnold (1999) argues that concepts of malaria and race were mutually constituted in colonial Bengal. Michael Worboys (1999) traces concepts of racial immunity to diseases such as tuberculosis.

In these discourses, hygiene and health became targets of research and intervention through colonists' interest in maintaining or increasing productivity and in their fears about contamination and epidemics that involved classifications of purity/impurity. These approaches also involved emerging scientific concepts. For example, Mark Jackson (1999) shows that the mentally ill were racialized and that races were understood in terms of emerging psychiatric deficiencies. These analyses argue that colonial encounters deeply integrated disease, health, and medicine in concepts of race.

6. As Worboys (1999: 158) shows, such race genetics was at times generative of research on particular conditions, as in the case of one colonial researcher working on tuberculosis in 1932: "[He] drew support from the new British and American studies on pathological and tissue differences between blacks and whites that were said to point to 'a true genotypic difference between the two races.'"

7. I restrict the following discussion to arguments about the physiological basis for race. I thereby elide the sophisticated critiques of the broader significance of race by critical theorists such as W. E. B. Du Bois, Frantz Fanon, and Franz Boas's students such as Ruth Benedict. (Faye Harrison [1995] points out that Du Bois also conducted physiological research to obviate direct associations between mental and physical attributes.) My restriction is meant to illustrate the traditions of arguments over precisely what is currently debated in the pages of the *New England Journal of Medicine, Journal of the American Medical Association, Nature,* and other medical and scientific journals. For a review of anthropological approaches to race over time, see Stocking 1982.

8. Ashley Montagu (1963b) argued the problematics in racial classification due to the gradations—the lack of purity—of any particular set of characteristics between groups. He also directed attention to the relational distinctions of race through critiques of the terms "Caucasian," "Mongoloid," and other groupings. His concept of "ethnic group" was designed to replace the term "race" in order to indicate the intermixture of the cultural and the biological in such groups (p. 1352).

9. In his response to Dobzhansky, Frank Livingstone (1962: 280) stressed what he considered their more fundamental disagreement: "To Dobzhansky races and race differences are things which exist 'out there' as biological phenomena, but race is also a label by which we describe 'out there.' I disagree. No science can divorce its concepts, definitions, and theories so completely from its subject matter, so that Dobzhansky's dichotomy between biological and nomenclatorial problems is impossible."

10. This discussion is significantly linked to the availability of the technologies and testing. The existence of a genetic test for a disease, or data suggestive of an ethnically specific drug response, create an ethical need as access to testing becomes a moral necessity. Troy Duster (2003) discusses an example of this process with Tay-Sachs disease, and the widespread interest in genetic testing among Jewish communities in the United States. Thus, where little interest or social attention may have been invested in genetic research toward a community, once such a test is manufactured or data created, the moral and social need becomes acute and can result in political and legal action. In this sense, the trajectory of genetics of race and disease and drug response can itself be generative of the moral need for the research.

11. I thank Carolyn Rouse for directing me to this article.

12. In nineteenth-century scientific studies, the table was used to organize race. The first systematic classifications of race are usually attributed to Johann Friedrich Blumenbach or Georges Cuvier (see, e.g., Stepan 1982; Augstein 1999; Banton 2000) Races, like

other living beings, were considered to have an internal logic that dictated their body type, behavior, and sociality. Such an approach could be seen in the pre-nineteenth-century discourse on race; what Cuvier created differently was a synthesis by which the table—a grid of physical similarities and differences—becomes the basis for understanding this internal logic. As a result, individual physical characteristics—measured with an increasing array of techniques and tools—were selected as representing the trajectory of each race. This move inverted the pre-nineteenth-century temporality of human variation: the variable contexts and experiences that had shaped bodies and physical attributes were now a background revealing the rigidity of the internal processes that shaped the progress of each race. Races differed radically in their internal mechanisms and had internal histories, making their temporalities more distinct from each other. Foucault (2003) and Stepan (1982) argue that in the nineteenth century, evolution shifted the meaning of history of races to adaptive characteristics and struggle between contiguous groups. Evolution was deployed by physical anthropologists to argue that other races were inferior in this struggle, and social evolutionism was used to place different races on hierarchies of progress, civilization, intelligence, spirituality, and other valued characteristics (Stepan 1982). My claim here is that in biomedicine and much of the biosciences, the table continues to be a more salient way of organizing knowledge about race than is the history used by geneticists exploring the evolution of human diversity; in biomedicine, this history tends to be incidentally added on to existing classifications rather than generative of new ones (on the use of speculation about evolution in biomedical approaches to race, see Kaufman and Hall 2003).

13. In an interview for the *New York Times Magazine,* Troy Duster offers an eloquent criticism of the attention on a future of individualized medicine: "The mantra of pharmacogenomics is that drugs will be fine-tuned for the individual. But individuals are not a market. Groups are a market" (Henig 2004: 49).

14. Jenny Reardon (2005) discusses a similar emphasis on a moral need to account for genetic diversity by population among the geneticists involved in the Human Genome Diversity Project (HGDP). However, whereas the HGDP group emphasized collection to preserve vanishing genetic information, the asthma geneticists focus on the disease disparities between different races.

15. James Boon (1999) cites James Clifford in this insight.

Chapter 2. The Nation as Biomedical Site

1. All names used, excluding those of cited authors, are pseudonyms. Where identifying information is included, names are excluded altogether. Unfortunately, in order to keep anonymity between groups of people I interacted with, I found I could not offer extended portrayals of these individuals in these pages: this fact at times ironically creates a depersonalization in my attempt to invoke personhood.

2. According to one AstraZeneca representative I spoke with, Symbicort had not yet been submitted for FDA approval because of marketing considerations (the company was focusing on Nexium, which would be followed by Crestor).

3. Veena Das and Deborah Poole (2004: 14) write about individuals who are simultaneously within and outside of the state: "It is precisely because they also act as representatives of the state that they are able to move across—and thus muddy—the seeming clear divide separating legal and extralegal forms of punishment and enforcement."

Here, I approach the pharmaceutical multinational as such an actor for the Drug Service committee members.

4. Don Robotham (1996) argues that the IMF is less influential in the Caribbean now than it was in the 1970s because the international market is a better enforcer of policies of deregulation, privatization, and trade liberalization. I am similarly arguing that rather than explicit policy, the interpretations and representations of global market practices and international institutional goals influence national policy.

5. This reduction is in locally produced pesticides. Use of imported pesticides has increased.

6. Robotham (1996: 308) argues that such analyses of international practices are foundational to Caribbean identities: "Identities in the Caribbean...tend to formulate themselves in the guise of some form of transnationalism, with social and economic issues coming rapidly to the forefront, seeking to contest the forces of globalization and transnationalization on the terrain of globalization itself, contesting modernity on the terrain of modernity."

Chapter 3. Asthma Variations

1. This brief sketch of the history of asthma relies primarily on historical research I conducted at the National Library of Medicine in addition to the work of Carla Keirns, and her dissertation on the history of asthma (2004). I thank Angela Creager for pointing me toward Carla Keirns's work.

2. John Floyer's approach reflected the focus on symptoms that historians have associated with medical understandings in the eighteenth century. According to Michel Foucault (1994b: 90;) "The symptom—hence its uniquely privileged position—is the form in which the disease is presented: of all that is visible, it is closest to the essential; it is the first transcription of the inaccessible nature of the disease. Cough, fever, pain in the side, and difficulty in breathing are not pleurisy itself—the disease itself is never exposed to the senses, but 'reveals itself only to reasoning'—but they form its 'essential symptoms.'" The essence of the disease in this medical perspective is hidden, according to Foucault, a kind of irreducible mystery of which the symptoms are the clues. In Floyer's account, wheezing and bronchial constriction were tied to the pulse as objects that reveal the disease: these were the visible forms of the underlying condition.

3. Foucault (1994b: 138) writes, "In other words, medical experience will substitute the *localization of the fixed point for the recording of frequencies.*"

4. Jan Sapp (1983) shows that what was called Mendelian heredity during the late nineteenth century existed within a context of multiple disciplinary approaches to heredity. Investigators in natural history (including paleontology, morphology, and others) examined visible characteristics of organisms to find their similarities and differences as evidence of their evolutionary history; cytologists focused on the physical aspect of heredity; embryologists included heredity within the process of development; for biometry, heredity was explained through statistical representation of changes at a species-wide level. Mendelian researchers, by differentiating organisms based on distribution of visible characteristics, offered one approach among many to understanding heredity in this context (1983).

5. To explain the medical details: response to medication is measured by conducting spirometry before and after the individual inhales a short-acting β_2 agonist; response

to methacholine is measured by conducting spirometry periodically as an individual inhales solutions with increasing levels of methacholine.

6. For asthma, in which response to medication is a common diagnostic technique, the line between pharmacogenetics and genetics of disease is often blurred. For example, DeCODE heralded its discovery of "a major susceptibility gene for asthma" as the basis to begin development of a pharmacogenomic test for inhaled steroids (DeCODE n.d.). Or research on genes for β2 adrenergic receptors (β2 AR) is used to explain both response to the β2 agonists and asthma severity (Rusnak et al. 2001; Hall 2001). More recently, the discovery of a gene that is thought to cause a predisposition to asthma, ADAM33, is being used to formulate new potential therapeutic targets.

7. Databases are at times centered around asthma, combining data and biological materials from different projects. Alternatively, the database can be focused on a population, as in DeCODE's Icelandic work, which is often discussed as the archetypal alternative large-scale whole-genome method to studying various diseases. Boundaries between academic and industry research are blurred in these collaborations but continue to have discursive function: pharmaceutical company representatives often portray academic research as insufficiently large scale to produce necessary data. Academic researchers portray industry work as insufficiently grounded in disease knowledge; that is, candidate gene approaches based on knowledge about disease mechanisms are valued as more informative than whole genome searches.

Chapter 4. (Re)Categorizing Asthma and the Rational Pharmaceutical

1. Barbadian health practitioners used differing measures to indicate high prevalence to me, including number of emergency room visits, self-reports of asthma, and amount of asthma medication taken, as is common in medical literature.

2. As James Boon (1990: xii) notes of anthropology, so too of biomedical science: "in disciplines like anthropology, 'the straight is crooked too,' and so is the crooked."

3. For families, the modernized diet brings polluted foods, as chemicals are included in the asthma-inducing changes wrought by modernization. Families particularly talked about chemicals brought into what they eat as a result of Barbados's place in the global economy (see chapter 6).

4. New Zealand and the United States accounted for more than half of the food imported to Barbados in 2001 (Barbados Statistical Service 2002b).

5. I do not want to give the impression that other ways of talking about asthma treatment preclude judgments of family behaviors: while I focus here on the most common discourse of adherence as intervention, discussion of prevention through environmental practices was also at times laden with rebuke. One pharmacist I talked with emphasized the need for such a focus because patients were taking advantage of the easy access to medications. He commented, "There's no real emphasis on prevention, there's no emphasis on taking responsibility for the disease."

6. Asthma education and outreach follow the radical individualization of biomedical representations found in current market systems (see Brandt 1997 and Beck 1999 for different analyses of this process of individualization; as Allan Brandt, and Charles Briggs (2005), note, such risk discourses carry moral prescriptions and proscriptions for individual and community behaviors). Pamphlets call for individualized treatment and the ethical imperatives of personalizing medical care. Asthma action plans attribute

responsibility to the individual—they describe causes of asthma attacks and techniques of intervention in terms of personal and family behaviors. This intervention is premised on population approaches. The design of inserts, the content of action plans, and the distribution of literature are based on remarkably extensive demographic research. The discourse of individualization is thereby importantly linked to the science of population analysis; indeed, it is statistical categorization of populations that engenders the discourse of individualization.

7. An interesting moral logic linking the pharmaceutical and tobacco industries was also posed during the lecture. The speaker talked about the tobacco industry as influential and causing the current increase in chronic obstructive pulmonary disease and possibly asthma, implying that the pharmaceutical company was a necessary counter to the tobacco industry.

Chapter 5. Biomedical Partnerships

1. For example, the success of the acute lung injury study was considered partially due to the presence of nurses at the six sites who could collect informed consent and data.

2. I thank Carol Greenhouse for this interpretation.

3. See Khan 2004 and Thomas 2004 for subtle explorations of the relationship of nationality and ethnicity in the Caribbean countries Trinidad and Jamaica, respectively. As Khan (2004: 41) argues, official discourses are themselves multiple in their approaches to race: "When Indians' context and point of reference is India, they are not 'white,' but they are 'Aryan,' they are 'Caucasian.' Caucasian/Aryan are associated with Brahmanical (that is, high culture) Hinduism. As indentured immigrants, however, they are even further from 'white,' becoming, as 'coolies,' increasingly 'black.'"

4. To put the case more biomedically, early underexpression of Th1, caused by decreased contact with pathogens and infections, results in overexpression of Th2, leading to increased sensitivity to allergens.

Chapter 6. Misgivings in Medical Participation

1. As Mary-Jo and Byron Good (2000) show, the use of new biomedicines and techniques entangles international and local meanings as the doctor-patient relationship produces the clinical narrative; illness experiences (Kleinman 1988) are given particular form as medical through this interaction. The restriction of the meaning of disease to etiology, in addition to systematically transforming or excluding the illness experience, also elides the lived experience of the lack of access or use of medicines, the problems and pains of hospital experiences, of blame from doctors, and of fear of medical systems, diagnostics, and treatments.

2. I thank Carol Greenhouse for helping me see this interpretation.

3. See Biehl et al. 2001 for an analysis of identity and disease around HIV-testing technologies.

4. These studies suggest that antibiotics given in childhood may cause asthma (for a review of this literature, see Marra et al. 2006).

5. See Orta 2004 for a recent subtle study in the relational distinction of global/local.

6. To use Lévi-Strauss's terms (1973), the *figurative consumption* of medications is valued in contrast to their *literal consumption*. This deferral of literal consumption is

a way of bringing the naturalized medical practice of prescribing pharmaceuticals into culture (able to be changed, manipulated, utilized to multiple ends).

7. Emily Martin and Richard Cone (n.d.) argue that the association of foreign foods with asthma may be supported by immunological evidence.

8. Frank and Alison thus critique the impact of the global economy on food production practices. As Sidney Mintz (1985) has shown, Barbados has historically been a primary site where the sugar industry has tied international food markets to Caribbean life through colonialism.

9. Frank's reference to chlordane implicates building materials in asthma; other families talked about asbestos in their home as a possible cause.

10. Following Lévi-Strauss (1966 and 1969) and Marilyn Strathern (1980), the nature/culture distinction is relational. In this sense, modern technologies, markets, and production can be sites of "nature." Lévi-Strauss argues that nature/culture distinctions are a means of organizing exchange systems. Objects are placed into one or the other domains in ways that reflect domestication and identify group boundaries. Objects that move across the nature/culture distinction are used to make meaning out of apparently unalterable or reified processes. By moving them into the domestic/cultural sphere, the process is placed into the world of human practice, allowing intervention, manipulation, and use.

11. I thank João Biehl for helping me see this interpretation.

Chapter 7. Participant Mothers

1. For an analysis of the shift in Barbadian economy and women workers, see Freeman 2000. She notes that the extended family as social network is a decreasing practice in Barbados. This trend exacerbates the problem of mother as individualized caretaker of the asthmatic.

2. As Carla Freeman (2000: 76) argues, this has produced contradictory ideals of womanhood: "The tasks of generating an income, managing the household, and having responsibility for child care all fell on women's shoulders in the absence of their men. These processes, together with women's longer history as a vital source of physical labor on the plantation, helped to establish what would become coexisting, and to some degree, contradictory, gender ideologies valuing domesticity and housewifery and the expectation of women's labor."

Chapter 8. Home Visit Translations

1. Usually a methacholine challenge would also be conducted using this technology. During the year that I did fieldwork, the team had decided not to include methacholine challenge because of the controversy surrounding the death of a participant in a Johns Hopkins asthma study.

2. For example: Anthropologist Aisha Khan (2004: 7) draws attention to analyses showing that the success of Portuguese colonialism was used in the Caribbean to code Portuguese as Europeans whose "whiteness" was more "negro" than the "colored" or "browns" who formed the middle class. She also shows that Indo-Trinidadian and Afro-Trinidadian Muslims have been ethnically linked, in contrast to both Indo-Trinidadian Hindus and Afro-Trinidadian Christians. Anthropologist Kay Warren (2001) notes that in Guatemala a shared Mayan language has been used to forge racial identities in contrast

to a hybrid mestizaje elite, in opposition to established claims of racial homogeneity. Sociologist Wolfgang Gabbert (2004) argues that in the mid-nineteenth century, Ladino prisoners on the Yucatan Peninsula formed an ethnic identity with descendants of Chinese laborers and descendants of black laborers in contrast to neighboring Maya-speaking peoples, in opposition to government discourses of a Mayan race. Historian Jeffrey Lesser (1999) argues that in Brazil, descendants of Japanese immigrants have historically been coded alternately as white in contrast to other populations in Brazil at some times and as racially connected to Brazilian indigenous populations at other times. Anthropologist Deborah James (1999) argues that in South Africa migrant women have created an identity category of Sotho ethnicity in contrast to the ethnic claims of Sotho men. Anthropologist Kevin Avruch (2002: 75) writes that in the Sudan, "'black'...northern (Muslim, Arabophone) Sudanese know themselves to be Arabs, and thus utterly different from the African (i.e. 'black') southern (Christian, non-Arabophone) Sudanese, with whom they have struggled in a bloody civil war for more than two decades now." Racial categorizations are contingently imbricated with gender, class, religion, and other means of drawing distinctions.

3. This contrasts with other links of nationhood and race: Don Robotham (1996) argues that prior to the 1960s, the identity of "West Indian" was a way of disassociating Caribbean people from black Americans and Africans. As Karen Olwig (1999) argues, discourses of Africa and history in the Caribbean today enact claims to political authority, responding particularly to changes wrought by tourism. H. Hoetnik (1985) reminds us that such analyses are largely restricted to the English-speaking Caribbean. Paul Gilroy (1993b) argues for the utility of black identities linking Caribbean, British, and North American peoples.

4. In my experience, Bajan medical practitioners emphasized the ethnic heterogeneity of Trinidad in particular. Aisha Khan's (1993) and Daniel Segal's (1993) works analyze the common Caribbean and Caribbeanist discourse constituting Trinidad as a "mix." Each explores ambiguity by focusing on where "mixing" and "coloured" are emphasized and where they are erased in the relational meanings of race.

As Khan (2004) argues, in Trinidadian discourses, a dichotomy of Indo-Trinidadian and Afro-Trinidadian sits uneasily with an ideology of a heterogeneous and mixed nation, all of which is further contested by the religious identities of Christian, Muslim, and Hindu. Khan nicely works through this multiplicity of identities while attending to the cultural construction of Trinidad as "multiple."

Segal offers a subtle summary of the ways racial categorizations are relational in Trinidad. The attributes of white in the distinction contrasting whites with Africans are different from the attributes of white in the distinction contrasting white and African with Indian: "In analyzing the meaning of *creole* in Trinidadian society of both the pre- and postindependence eras, my earlier work argued that the simultaneous hyperrecognition of 'European'-'African' mixing and hyporecognition of 'European'-'Indian' mixing were determined by contrastive racial typifications of 'Orientals' and 'Africans.' 'The Oriental,' I argued, was typified as saturated, to her or his very core, by a distinct and inert (or 'ancient') civilizational character. 'The African' by contrast, was typified as civilizationally naked and—almost redundantly—as stripped by the Middle Passage of even the minimal trappings of culture that, it was imagined, were all that was present in the ancestral homeland of Africa. By these contrastive racial typifications (which can also be recognized as contrastive principles of subordination), 'the African' possessed an excess of miscibilty, whereas 'the Indian' was constructed as stubbornly resistant to 'mixing.'" (2006: 580). In this reading, hybridity and tendency toward hybridity are considered a characteristic of one racial type, making it categorically distinct from the associated tendency toward purity of another. Segal's work has long been attuned to the ways in racial categorizations—not only are the categories relational but so are the relations between categories.

5. Bill Maurer (2000) discusses a similar multiplicity among British Virgin Islander notions of ethnicity.

6. As Shalini Puri (2003) points out, such carnivals, even while opening up, playing with, and rejecting some established hierarchies, also maintain, bolster, and entrench others. Where Puri argues for the significance of attending to this dialectic in any analysis of Carnival, I am less optimistic about the possibility of a fully comprehensive approach. I consider analytic emphases on the subversions accomplished by Carnival to contain as much possibility for intricate innovations as emphases on the relationship of hierarchies criticized and hierarchies maintained, which Puri's analyses are so adept at (e.g., see her insights on the play of ambivalence in Carnival spectacles about Trinidad's transnational connections with the United States).

7. Lundy Braun (2005) shows that this use of statistical techniques and technological measurements shaped gendered and racialized meanings of asthma in the nineteenth century. During the Civil War, the spirometer, which measured "vital capacity" according to its originator, was employed in studies of Union soldiers. (Braun shows that the term "vital capacity" was itself tied to concepts of progress, industrialization, and labor welfare in nineteenth-century England.) The result was a stratification of races according to their vital capacity: Braun argues that this formulation was the origin of the current common practice of adjusting asthma measurements for race. I thank Duana Fullwiley for introducing me to Braun's work.

8. This evaluation of the technology—as arcane, strange, and associated with expertise—was relational: the Barbadian study facilitators also considered this technology to be complex and require explanation and interpretation. The study facilitators and I would go to a Barbadian leptospirosis laboratory after each day of home visits. There the tubes of blood would be spun on a centrifuge as preparation for storage, until they could be shipped from that lab to the United States for analysis by the geneticists. During the time I spent in Barbados, the centrifuge, spirometer, and computer programs required several negotiations about calibration and use between lab technicians, geneticists, and study facilitators. Data analysis also required differing levels of expertise, as clinicians, epidemiologists, and population geneticists brought particular approaches to the team. Each of these experts invested meaning into the others' technologies and analyses, as authoritative, significant to asthma meaning, and opaque: in these interactions, the science of population genetics could be as arcane to clinicians as lung response was to the geneticist. Biomedical science, like other ways of knowing, includes the use of objects arcane and unknown to the user.

9. When one study facilitator asked about this policy, one of the genetics team members noted that without genetic counselors, it would be improper for the team to give genetic results.

10. The allergen test was currently available from one immunologist in Barbados at a cost prohibitive to almost all of the participants in the asthma study.

11. The allergen test thereby performs a mediatory function, in Lévi-Strauss's sense: the test operates to link different levels of symbolic relations (see particularly Lévi-Strauss

1990: 469). The allergen test, at one level, provides a disjunction between the participant and other Bajan asthmatics (as an extra form of intervention not found elsewhere in Barbados). On the symbolic level of genetics and the patient experience, the test operates as a conjunction (as incorporating the arcane of genetics into the lived experience of the illness). And these levels include the ambivalence toward U.S.-based funding and technologies, international markets, and medical practice defining disease.

12. For discussion of hybridity as multiple, vernacular, and constitutive, see Gilroy 1993a; Bhabha 1994; Boon 1998. Recent anthropological literature on Latin America and on the Caribbean has criticized overly simple uses of hybridity in cultural criticism (see Khan 2001; Rahier 2003; Alonso 2004; Puri 2004; Munasinghe 2006). These authors point to the ways official discourses that value hybridity (mestizaje, mixing, callaloo, creole) are used to marginalize disadvantaged populations, and the way analytic emphases on hybridity can inadvertently instantiate purities. As Khan (2004: 17 18) points out, when "mixed" becomes a means of distinguishing some people, or language, or nation from another, it becomes yet another purity: "[Afro-Trinidadian versus Indo-Trinidadian is a] racial divide as neat and precise as its counterimage, the mixed and imbricated callaloo nation." I here emphasize Boon's, Bhabha's, and Gilroy's interest in hybridity as vernacular, as foundationally multiple. The point here is to remain attentive to the irreducibility of narratives and practices to any posited actual political economy, history, or even discourse. What these authors are championing is not any use of hybridity anywhere, but rather hybridity as a refusal to accept any purity. It is exceedingly difficult to determine if any uses of hybridity avoid this trap, but this is part of the paradox of trying to offer a *representation* of *representations*. That is to say, how are we to speak of multiplicity without reducing it to a (single) thing?

Chapter 9. Biomedical and Anthropological Excesses

1. Scientific practice is cultural like George Steiner's notion of human speech (1998: 213): "But it is its great untidiness that makes human speech innovative and expressive of personal intent. It is the anomaly, as it feeds back into the general history of usage, the ambiguity, as it enriches and complicates the general standard of definition, which gives coherence to the system. A coherence, if such a description is allowed, 'in constant motion.'" The moments of ambivalence are akin to the anomalous objects that reveal play with cultural categories: the oral steroids and allergen tests for the families, the gene-environment study for geneticists, reveal the slippage and critique inherent in the efficacy of discursive systems.

2. Gregory Bateson (2000) and Claude Lévi-Strauss (1963) draw attention to such operations. In Bateson's writing on the alcoholic (2000: 311), the individual's contradictory self-conceptions reinforce each other: "The present theory of alcoholism, therefore, will provide a *converse matching* between the sobriety and the intoxication, such that the latter may be seen as an appropriate subjective correction for the former." Lévi-Strauss similarly finds an integrated contradiction in two alternate explanations for an event of sorcery held by a group of native Brazilians that he lived among. He (1963: 169) writes, "The important point is that these two possibilities were not mutually exclusive; no more than are, for us, the alternate interpretations of war as the dying gasp of national independence or as the result of the schemes of munitions manufacturers. The two explanations are logically incompatible, but we admit that one or the other may be true;

since they are equally plausible, we easily make the transition from one to the other, depending on the occasion and the moment. Many people have both explanations in the back of their minds."

3. As Jean Pouillon (1982: 5) writes, "Ambiguity is not simply polysemy, the fact that a verb sometimes has one meaning and sometimes another, each of them unequivocal; it is, rather, that, above all, there is always doubt at the heart of the conviction, and that the affirmation itself indicates that it could always be suspended."

4. Lévi-Strauss (1981: 603) writes, "It cannot be said purely and simply of the world that it is: it exists in the form of an initial asymmetry, which shows itself in a variety of ways according to the angle from which it is being apprehended: between the high and the low, the sky and the earth, land and water, the near and the far, left and right, male and female, etc."

5. As Clarice Lispector (1988: 101)writes, "If 'truth' were what I can understand…it would end up being but a small truth, my-sized. Truth must reside precisely in what I shall never understand."

References

Ahmadi, Kourosh R., and David B. Goldstein. 2002. "Multifactorial Diseases: Asthma Genetics Point the Way." *Current Biology* 12: 702–4.

Alonso, Ana Maria. 2004. "Conforming Disconformity: 'Mestizaje,' Hybridity, and the Aesthetics of Mexican Nationalism." *Cultural Anthropology* 19(4): 459–90.

Anderlik, Mary R., and Mark A. Rothstein. 2001. "Privacy and Confidentiality of Genetic Information: What Rules for the New Science?" *Annual Review of Genomic and Human Genetics* 2: 401–33.

Angell, Marcia. 2004. *The Truth about Drug Companies: How They Deceive Us and What to Do about It.* New York: Random House.

Apter, Andrea J., Susan T. Reisine, Glenn Affleck, Erik Barrows, and Richard L. Zu-Wallack. 1998. "Adherence with Twice-Daily Dosing of Inhaled Steroids: Socioeconomic and Health-Belief Differences." *American Journal of Respiratory and Critical Care Medicine* 157(6): 1810–17.

Arnold, David. 1999. "'An Ancient Race Outworn': Malaria and Race in Colonial India, 1860–1930." In *Race, Science, and Medicine, 1700–1960,* ed. Waltraud Ernst and Bernard Harris, 123–43. New York: Routledge.

Augstein, H. F. 1999. "From the Land of the Bible to the Caucasus and Beyond: The Shifting Ideas of the Geographical Origin of Humankind." In *Race, Science, and Medicine, 1700–1960,* ed. Waltraud Ernst and Bernard Harris, 58–79. New York: Routledge.

Avruch, Kevin. 2002. "Culture and Ethnic Conflict in the New World Disorder." In *Race and Ethnicity: Comparative and Theoretical Approaches,* ed. John Stone and Rutledge Dennis, 72–82. Oxford: Blackwell.

Banton, Michael. 2000. "The Idiom of Race: A Critique of Presentism." In *Theories of Race and Racism*, ed. Les Back and John Solomos, 51–63. New York: Routledge.

Barbados Statistical Service. 2002a. *2000 Population and Housing Census*. Barbados: Barbados Statistical Service.

———. 2002b. *Annual Overseas Trade 2001*. Barbados: Barbados Statistical Service.

Barnes, Kathleen C., Rasika A. Mathias, Renate Nickel, Linda R. Freidhoff, Maria L. Stockton, Xielen Xue, Raana P. Naidu, Paul N. Levett, Vincenzo Casolaro, and Terri H. Beaty. 2001. "Testing for Gene-Gene Interaction Controlling Total IgE in Families from Barbados: Evidence of Sensitivity regarding Linkage Heterogeneity among Families." *Genomics* 71: 246–51.

Barnes, Kathleen C., John D. Neely, David L. Duffy, Linda R. Freidhoff, Daniel R. Breazeale, Carsten Schou, Raana P. Naidu, Paul N. Levett, Beatrice Renault, Raju Kucherlapati, Sebastiano Iozzino, Eva Ehrlich, Terri H. Beaty, and David G. Marsh. 1996. "Linkage of Asthma and Total Serum IgE Concentration to Markers on Chromosome 12Q: Evidence from Afro-Caribbean and Caucasian Populations." *Genomics* 37: 41–50.

Barrow, Christine. 1999 [1996]. *Family in the Caribbean: Themes and Perspectives*. Princeton: Markus Weiner.

Bateson, Gregory. 1958 [1936]. *Naven (2nd ed.)*. Palo Alto, CA: Stanford University Press.

———. 2000 [1972]. "The Cybernetics of 'Self': A Theory of Alcoholism." In *Steps to an Ecology of Mind*, 309–37. Chicago: University of Chicago Press.

Beck, Ulrich. 1992. *Risk Society: Towards a New Modernity*. London: Sage Press.

———. 1999. *World Risk Society*. Malden, MA: Polity Press.

Beckles, Hilary. 1990. *A History of Barbados: From Amerindian Settlement to Nation-State*. Cambridge: Cambridge University Press.

Bender, Bruce G. 2002. "Overcoming Barriers to Nonadherence in Asthma Treatment." *Journal of Allergy and Clinical Immunology* 109(6 Suppl.): S554–59.

Berkart, J. B. 1916. *The Pathology and Treatment of the So-Called Nervous Asthma*. New York: Oxford University Press.

Bhabha, Homi K. 1994. "'Race,' Time and the Revision of Modernity." In *The Location of Culture*, 338–67. New York: Routledge.

Biehl, João. 2004a. "The Activist State: Global Pharmaceuticals, AIDS, and Citizenship in Brazil." *Social Text* 80, 22(3): 105–32.

———. 2004b. "Life of the Mind: The Interface of Psychopharmaceuticals, Domestic Economies, and Social Abandonment." *American Ethnologist* 31(4): 475–96.

Biehl, João, Denise Coutinho, and Ana Luzia Outeiro. 2001. "Technology and Affect: HIV/AIDS Testing in Brazil." *Culture, Medicine, and Psychiatry* 25(1): 87–129.

Blumenthal, Malcom N., Carl D. Langefeld, Terri H. Beaty, Eugene R. Bleecker, Carole Ober, Lucille Lester, Ethan Lange, Kathleen C. Barnes, Raoul Wolf, Richard A. King, Julian Solway, William Oetting, Deborah A. Meyers, and Stephen S. Rich. 2003. "A Genome-Wide Search for Allergic Response (Atopy) Genes in Three Ethnic Groups: Collaborative Study on the Genetics of Asthma." *Human Genetics* 112(5–6): 600–609.

Boas, Franz. 1983. *The Mind of Primitive Man*. Westport, CT: Greenwood Press.

Boon, James A. 1980. "Comparative De-enlightenment: Paradox and Limits in the History of Ethnology." *Daedalus* 109(2): 73–91.

———. 1982. *Other Tribes, Other Scribes: Symbolic Anthropology in the Comparative Study of Cultures, Histories, Religions, and Texts.* New York: Cambridge University Press.

———. 1990. *Affinities and Extremes: Crisscrossing the Bittersweet Ethnology of East Indies History, Balinese Culture, and Indo-European Allure.* Chicago: University of Chicago Press.

———. 1998. "Accenting Hybridity: Postcolonial Cultural Studies, a Boasian Anthropologist, and I." In *'Culture' and the Problem of the Disciplines,* ed. John Carlos Rowe, 141–70. New York: Columbia University Press.

———. 1999. *Verging on Extra-Vagance: Anthropology, History, Religion, Literature, Arts... Showbiz.* Princeton: Princeton University Press.

Brace, C. L. 1964. "On the Race Concept." *Current Anthropology* 5(4): 313–20.

Brandt, Allan M. 1997. "Behavior, Disease, and Health in the Twentieth-Century United States: The Moral Valence of Risk." In *Morality and Health,* ed. Allan M. Brandt and Paul Rozin, 53–77. New York: Routledge.

Braun, Lundy. 2002. "Race, Ethnicity, and Health: Can Genetics Explain Disparities?" *Perspectives in Biology and Medicine* 45(2): 159–74.

———. 2005. "Spirometry, Measurement, and Race in the Nineteenth Century." *Journal of the History of Medicine and Allied Sciences* 60(2): 135–69.

Braun, Lundy, Anne Fausto-Sterling, Duana Fullwiley, Evelyn M. Hammonds, Alondra Nelson, William Quivers, Susan M. Reverby, Alexandra E. Shields. 2007. "Racial Categories in Medical Practice: How Useful Are They?" *PLoS Medicine* 4(9)e271: 1423–28.

Bray, George William. 1931. *Recent Advances in Allergy (Asthma, Hay-Fever, Eczema, Migraine, etc).* Philadelphia: P. Blakiston's.

Bree, Robert. 1797. *A Practical Inquiry on Disordered Respiration: Distinguishing the Species of Convulsive Asthma, Their Causes, and Indications of Cure.* Birmingham: G. G. and J. Robinson.

Briggs, Charles L. 2005. "Communicability, Racial Discourse, and Disease." *Annual Review of Anthropology* 34: 269–91.

Bulmer, Ralph. 1970 [1967]. "Why the Cassowary Is Not a Bird." In *Rules and Meanings: The Anthropology of Everyday Knowledge,* ed. Mary Douglas, 167–93. Hammondsworth, England: Penguin Education.

Califano, Andrea, Ned McCullough, Allen Buchanan, Elizabeth McPherson, Baruch A. Brody, Jeffrey Kahn, and John A. Robertson. 2002. "Pharmacogenetics: Ethical and Regulatory Issues in Research and Clinical Practice: Report of the Consortium on Pharmacogenetics: Findings and Recommendations." Unpublished manuscript. Minneapolis, MN: The Consortium on Pharmacogenetics.

Centers for Disease Control and Prevention. 2002. "Self-Reported Increase in Asthma Severity after the September 11 Attacks on the World Trade Center—Manhattan, New York." *Journal of the American Medical Association* 288(12): 1466–67.

Committee on Understanding and Eliminating Racial and Ethnic Disparities in Health Care. 2002. "Introduction and Literature Review." In *Unequal Treatment: Confronting*

Racial and Ethnic Disparities in Health Care, ed. Brian D. Smedley, Adrienne Y. Stith, and Alan E. Nelson, 29–79. Washington, DC: National Academies Press.

Cooke, Robert A., and Albert Vander Veer. 1913. "Human Sensitization." *Journal of Immunology* 1: 201–18.

Coon, Carleton S. 1964. "Comment on 'On the Race Concept.'" *Current Anthropology* 5(4): 314.

Count, Earl W. 1964. "Comment on 'On the Race Concept.'" *Current Anthropology* 5(4): 314–16.

Das, Veena. 1998. "Wittgenstein and Anthropology." *Annual Review of Anthropology* 27: 171–95.

Das, Veena, and Ranendra K. Das. 2006. "Pharmaceuticals in Urban Ecologies: The Register of the Local." In *Global Pharmaceuticals: Ethics, Markets, Practices,* ed. Adriana Petryna, Andrew Lakoff, and Arthur Kleinman, 171–205. Durham: Duke University Press.

———. 2007. "How the Body Speaks: Illness and the Lifeworld among the Urban Poor." In *Subjectivity: Ethnographic Investigations,* ed. João Biehl, Arthur Kleinman, and Byron Good, 66–97. Berkeley, CA: University of California Press.

Das, Veena, and Deborah Poole. 2004. "State and Its Margins: Comparative Ethnographies." In *Anthropology in the Margins of the State,* ed. Veena Das and Deborah Poole, 3–34. Santa Fe: School of American Research Press.

DeCODE. n.d. "Press Releases." www.decode.com.

Dobzhansky, Theodosius. 1962. "Reply to 'On the Non-existence of Human Races.'" *Current Anthropology* 3(3): 280–81.

Douglas, Mary. 1966. *Purity and Danger.* New York: Praeger.

Dunwell, Patricia, and Arlene Rose. 2003. "Study of the Skin Disease Spectrum Occurring in an Afro-Caribbean Population." *International Journal of Dermatology* 42: 287–89.

Duster, Troy. 2003 [1990]. *Backdoor to Eugenics* (2nd ed.). New York: Routledge.

———. 2005. "Buried Alive: The Concept of Race in Science." In *Genetic Nature/ Culture: Anthropology and Science Beyond the Two Culture Divide.* Ed. Alan H. Goodman, Deborah Heath, and M. Susan Lindee, 258–77. Berkeley: University of California Press.

Eisner, Mark D., Patricia P. Katz, Edward H. Yelin, Stephen C. Shiboski, and Paul D. Blanc. 2000. "Risk Factors for Hospitalization among Adults with Asthma: The Influence of Sociodemographic Factors and Asthma Severity." *Respiratory Research* 2: 53–60.

Epstein, Steven. 1996. *Impure Science: AIDS, Activism, and the Politics of Knowledge.* Berkeley: University of California Press.

Ernst, Waltraud. 1999a. "Colonial Policies, Racial Politics and the Development of Psychiatric Institutions in Early Nineteenth Century British India." In *Race, Science, and Medicine, 1700–1960,* ed. Waltraud Ernst and Bernard Harris, 80–100. New York: Routledge.

———. 1999b. "Introduction: Historical and Contemporary Perspectives on Race, Science and Medicine." In *Race, Science, and Medicine, 1700–1960,* ed. Waltraud Ernst and Bernard Harris, 1–28. New York: Routledge.

Esteban, J. Parra, Amy Marcini, Joshua Akey, Jeremy Martinson, Mark A. Batzer, Richard Cooper, Terrence Forrester, David B. Allison, Ranjan Deka, Robert E. Ferrell, and Mark D. Shriver. 1998. "Estimating African American Admixture Proportions by Use of Population-Specific Alleles." *American Journal of Human Genetics* 63: 1839–51.

Exner, Derek V., Daniel L. Dries, Michael J. Domanski, and Jay N. Crohn. 2001. "Lesser Response to Angiotensin-Converting-Enzyme Inhibitor Therapy in Blacks as Compared with White Patients with Left Ventricular Dysfunction." *New England Journal of Medicine* 344(18): 1351–57.

Farmer, Paul. 2000. "The Consumption of the Poor: Tuberculosis in the 21st Century." *Ethnography* 1(2): 183–216.

Fenech, A., and Ian P. Hall. 2002. "Pharmacogenetics of Asthma." *British Journal of Clinical Pharmacology* 53: 2–15.

Fischer, Michael M. J. 2001. "Ethnographic Critique and Technoscientific Narratives: The Old Mole, Ethical Plateaux, and the Governance of Emergent Biosocial Politics." *Culture, Medicine, and Psychiatry* 25: 355–93.

Floyer, John. 1698. *A Treatise of the Asthma: Divided into Four Parts.* London: Printed for Richard Wilkin.

Food and Drug Administration. 2003. "Guidance for Industry: Collection of Race and Ethnicity Data in Clinical Trials." Unpublished pamphlet. Rockville, MD: U.S. Food and Drug Administration.

Fortun, Michael. 1998. "The Human Genome Project and the Acceleration of Biotechnology." In *Private Science: Biotechnology and the Rise of the Molecular Sciences,* ed. Arnold Thackray, 182–201. Philadelphia: University of Pennsylvania Press.

Foster, Morris W. 2003. "Pharmacogenomics and the Social Construction of Identity." In *Pharmacogenomics: Social, Ethical and Clinical Dimensions,* ed. Mark A. Rothstein, 251–66. Hoboken, NJ: John Wiley.

Foster, Morris W., and Richard R. Sharp. 2002. "Race, Ethnicity, and Genomics: Social Classifications as Proxies of Biological Heterogeneity." *Genome Research* 12(6): 844–50.

Foucault, Michel. 1994a [1970 Engl. trans.]. *The Order of Things: An Archaeology of the Human Sciences.* New York: Vintage.

———. 1994b [Engl. trans. 1973]. *The Birth of the Clinic: An Archaeology of Medical Perception.* New York: Vintage Books.

———. 2003 [1997]. *"Society Must Be Defended": Lectures at the College de France 1975–1976,* ed. Mauro Bertani and Alessandro Fontana, trans. David Macey. New York: Picador.

Freeman, Carla. 2000. *High Tech and High Heels in the Global Economy: Women, Work, and Pink-Collar Identities in the Caribbean.* Durham: Duke University Press.

Fuhlbrigge, Anne L., Robert J. Adams, Theresa W. Guilbert, Evie Grant, Paula Lozano, Susan L. Janson, Fernando Martinez, Kevin B. Weiss, and Scott T. Weiss. 2002. "The Burden of Asthma in the United States: Level and Distribution Are Dependent on the Interpretation of the NAEPP Guidelines." *American Journal of Respiratory and Critical Care Medicine* 166: 1044–49.

Fullwiley, Duana. n.d. Personal communication.

Gabbert, Wolfgang. 2004. "Of Friends and Foes: The Caste War and Ethnicity in Yucatan." *Journal of Latin American Anthropology* 9(1): 90–118.

Gaudillière, Jean-Paul, and Ilana Lwy. 2001. "Horizontal and Vertical Transmission of Diseases: The Impossible Separation." In *Heredity and Infection: The History of Disease Transmission*, ed. Jean-Paul Gaudillière and Ilana Lwy, 1–18. New York: Routledge.

Geertz, Clifford. 1973. "Thick Description: Toward an Interpretive Theory of Culture." In *The Interpretation of Cultures*, 3–30. New York: Basic Books.

Gilroy, Paul. 1993a. "It's a Family Affair: Black Culture and the Trope of Kinship." In *Small Acts: Thoughts on the Politics of Black Cultures*, 192–207. New York: Serpent's Tail.

———. 1993b. *The Black Atlantic: Modernity and Double Consciousness*. Cambridge: Harvard University Press.

Glauber, James H., and Anne L. Fuhlbrigge. 2002. "Stratifying Asthma Populations by Medication Use." *Annals of Allergy, Asthma, and Immunology* 88: 451–56.

Good, Mary-Jo DelVecchio. 2001. "The Biotechnical Embrace." *Culture, Medicine, and Psychiatry* (25): 395–410.

Good, Mary-Jo DelVecchio, and Byron Good. 2000. "Clinical Narratives and the Study of Contemporary Doctor-Patient Relationships." In *The Handbook of Social Studies in Health and Medicine*, ed. Gary L. Albrecht, Ray Fitzpatrick, and Susan C. Scrimshaw, 243–58. London: Sage Publications.

Good, Mary-Jo DelVecchio, Cara James, Byron Good, and Anne Becker. 2002. "The Culture of Medicine and Racial, Ethnic and Class Disparities in Health Care." In *Unequal Treatment: Confronting Racial and Ethnic Disparities in Health Care*, ed. Brian D. Smedley, Adrienne Y. Stith, and Alan E. Nelson, 594–625. Washington, DC: National Academies Press.

Goozner, Merrill. 2004. *The $800 Million Pill: The Truth behind the Cost of New Drugs*. Berkeley: University of California Press.

Gower, B. A., J. R. Fernandez, T. M. Beasley, M. D. Shriver, and M. I. Goran. 2003. "Using Genetic Admixture to Explain Racial Differences in Insulin-Related Phenotypes." *Diabetes* 52(4): 1047–51.

Grady, Denise. 2005. "Experts to Consider Withdrawal of Asthma Drugs." *New York Times* July 13.

Graves, Joseph L. 2001. *The Emperor's New Clothes*. New Brunswick, NJ: Rutgers University Press.

Greaves, Gaye, and Mary Jerrett. n.d. "An Asthma Education Programme and Evaluation with Primary School Children in Barbados." Unpublished manuscript. Queen Elizabeth Hospital, Barbados.

Gusterson, Hugh. 1996. *Nuclear Rites: A Weapons Laboratory at the End of the Cold War*. Berkeley: University of California Press.

Haga, Susanne B., and J. Craig Venter. 2003. "FDA Races in Wrong Direction." *Science* 301: 466.

Hall, Ian P. 2001. "Pharmacogenetics, Pharmacogenomics and Airway Disease." *Respiratory Research* 3(1): 10.

Hall, Percy. 1930. *Asthma and Its Treatment.* London: William Heinemann.

Hall, Stuart. 1997 [1991]. "Old and New Identities, Old and New Ethnicities." In *Culture, Globalization, and the World System: Contemporary Conditions for the Representation of Identity,* ed. Anthony D. King, 41–68. Minnesota: University of Minnesota Press.

Handler, Richard, and Daniel Segal. 1999 [1990]. *Jane Austen and the Fiction of Culture: An Essay on the Narration of Social Realities.* Lanham, MD: Rowman and Littlefield.

Haraway, Donna. 1997 *Modest_Witness@Second_Millenium.FemaleMan_Meets_On comouse.* New York: Routledge.

Harrison, Faye V. 1995. "The Persistent Power of 'Race' in the Cultural and Political Economy of Racism." *Annual Review of Anthropology* 24: 47–74.

Hedgecoe, Adam. 2004. *The Politics of Personalised Medicine: Pharmacogenetics in the Clinic.* Cambridge: Cambridge University Press.

Henig, Robin Marantz. 2004. "The Genome in Black and White (and Gray)." *New York Times Magazine* October 10.

Hoetnik, H. 1985. "'Race' and Color in the Caribbean." In *Caribbean Contours,* ed. Sidney W. Mintz and Sally Price, 55–84. Baltimore: Johns Hopkins University Press.

Huang, Shau-Ku, Rasika A. Mathias, Eva Ehrlich, Beverly Plunkett, Xin Liu, Garry R. Cutting, Xin-Jing Wang, Xiao-Dong Li, Alkis Togias, Kathleen C. Barnes, Floyd Malveaux, Stephen Rich, Beverly Mellen, Ethan Lange, Terri H. Beaty, and Comparative Study on the Genetics of Asthma. 2003. "Evidence for Asthma Susceptibility Genes on Chromosome 11 in an African-American Population." *Human Genetics* 113(1): 71–85.

Hunter, C. J., C. E. Brightling, G. Woltmann, A. J. Wardlaw, and I. D. Pavord. 2002. "A Comparison of the Validity of Different Diagnostic Tests in Adults with Asthma." *Chest* 121: 1051–57.

Hymes, Dell H. 1977. "The 'Wife' Who 'Goes out' Like a Man: Reinterpretation of a Clackamas Chinook Myth." In *Symbolic Anthropology: A Reader in the Study of Symbols and Meanings,* ed. Janet L. Dolgin, David S. Kemnitzer, and David M. Schneder, 221–44. New York: Columbia University Press.

International Monetary Fund. 2003. *IMF Report: Hard Choices to Be Made.* Washington, DC: International Monetary Fund.

———. 2004. *IMF Country Report No. 04/154: Barbados: 2004 Article IV Consultation—Staff Report; Public Information Notice on the Executive Board Discussion; and Statement by the Executive Director for Barbados.* Washington, DC: International Monetary Fund.

Issa, Amalia M. 2002. "Ethical Perspectives on Pharmacogenomic Profiling in the Drug Development Process." *Nature Reviews Drug Discovery* 1: 300–308.

Jackson, Mark. 1999. "Changing Depictions of Disease: Race, Representation, and the History of 'Mongolism.'" In *Race, Science, and Medicine, 1700–1960,* ed. Waltraud Ernst and Bernard Harris, 167–88. New York: Routledge.

James, Deborah. 1999. "Bagagešu (those of my home): Women Migrants, Ethnicity, and Performance in South Africa." *American Ethnologist* 26(1): 69–89.

Jones, David S., and Roy H. Perlis. 2006. "Pharmacogenetics, Race, and Psychiatry: Prospects and Challenges." *Harvard Review: Psychiatry* 14(2): 92–108.

Jones, James H. 1981. *Bad Blood: The Tuskegee Syphilis Experiment*. New York: Free Press.

Jorde, L. B., W. S. Watkins, and M. J. Bamshad. 2001. "Population Genomics: A Bridge from Evolutionary History to Genetic Medicine." *Human Molecular Genetics* 10(2): 2199–207.

Kahn, Jonathan. 2004. "How a Drug Becomes 'Ethnic': Law, Commerce, and the Production of Racial Categories in Medicine." *Yale Journal of Health Policy, Law, and Ethics* 4(1): 1–46.

Kamat, Vinay R., and Mark Nichter. 1998. "Pharmacies, Self-Medication and Pharmaceutical Marketing in Bombay, India." *Social Science and Medicine* 47(6): 779–94.

Kaplan, Martha, and John D. Kelly. 2000. "On Discourse and Power: 'Cults' and 'Orientals' in Fiji." *American Ethnologist* 26(4): 843–63.

Kaufman, Jay S., and Susan A. Hall. 2003. "The Slavery Hypertension Hypothesis: Dissemination and Appeal of a Modern Race Theory." *Epidemiology* 14(1): 111–18.

Kay, Lily E. 2000. *Who Wrote the Book of Life? A History of the Genetic Code*. Palo Alto, CA: Stanford University Press.

Keirns, Carla Christine. 2004. "Short of Breath: A Social and Intellectual History of Asthma in the United States." Ph.D. Dissertation, University of Pennsylvania.

Keller, Evelyn Fox. 1995. *Refiguring Life: Metaphors of Twentieth Century Biology*. New York: Columbia University Press.

Kevles, Daniel J. 1995 [1985]. *In the Name of Eugenics: Genetics and the Uses of Human Heredity*. Cambridge: Harvard University Press.

Khan, Aisha. 1993. "What Is a 'Spanish'?: Ambiguity and 'Mixed' Ethnicity in Trinidad." In *Trinidad Ethnicity*, ed. Kevin Yelvington, 180–207. Knoxville: University of Tennessee Press.

———. 2001. "Journey to the Center of the Earth: The Caribbean as Master Symbol." *Cultural Anthropology* 16(3): 271–302.

———. 2004. *Callaloo Nation: Metaphors of Race and Religious Identity among South Asians in Trinidad*. Durham: Duke University Press.

Kingscote, Ernest. 1899. *Asthma: Recent Development in Its Treatment*. London: Henry J. Glaisher.

Kleinman, Arthur. 1988. *The Illness Narratives: Suffering, Healing, and Human Experience*. New York: Basic Books.

Kousta, E., N. J. Lawrence, V. Anyaoku, D. G. Johnston, and M. I. McCarthy. 2001. "Prevalence and Features of Pancreatic Islet Cell Autoimmunity in Women with Gestational Diabetes from Different Ethnic Groups." *British Journal of Obstetrics and Gynaecology* 108: 716–20.

Lakoff, Andrew. 2006. "High Contact: Gifts and Surveillance in Argentina." In *Global Pharmaceuticals: Ethics, Markets, Practices*, ed. Adriana Petryna, Andrew Lakoff, and Arthur Kleinman, 111–35. Durham: Duke University Press.

Lang, David M., and Marcia Polansky. 1994. "Patterns of Asthma Mortality in Philadelphia from 1969 to 1991." *New England Journal of Medicine* 331(2): 1542–46.

Latour, Bruno. 1999. "Give Me a Laboratory and I Will Raise the World." In *The Science Studies Reader*, ed. Mario Biagioli, 258–75. New York: Routledge.

Latour, Bruno, and Steve Woolgar. 1979. *Laboratory Life: The Social Construction of Scientific Facts*. Beverly Hills: Sage.

Lee, Sandra Soo-Jin, Joanna Mountain, and Barbara A. Koenig. 2001. "The Meanings of 'Race' in the New Genomics: Implications for Health Disparities Research." *Yale Journal of Health Policy, Law, and Ethics* 1: 33–75.

Lesser, Jeffrey. 1999. *Negotiating National Identity: Immigrants, Minorities, and the Struggle for Ethnicity in Brazil*. Durham: Duke University Press.

Lester, Lucille A., Stephen S. Rich, Malcolm N. Blumenthal, Alkis Togias, Shirley Murphy, Floyd Malveaux, Michael E. Miller, Georgia M. Dunston, Julian Solway, Raoul L. Wolf, Jonathan M. Samet, David G. Marsh, Deborah A. Meyers, Carole Ober, Eugene R. Bleecker, and the Collaborative Study on the Genetics of Asthma. 2001. "Ethnic Differences in Asthma and Associated Phenotypes: Collaborative Study on the Genetics of Asthma." *Journal of Allergy and Clinical Immunology* 108(3): 357–62.

Lévi-Strauss, Claude. 1963 (Engl. trans.). "The Sorcerer and His Magic." In *Structural Anthropology*, trans. Clair Jacobson and Brooke Grundfest Schoepf, 167–85. New York: Basic Books.

———. 1966 (Engl. trans.). *The Savage Mind*. Chicago: University of Chicago Press.

———. 1969 (Engl. trans.). *The Elementary Structures of Kinship*. James Harle Bell, John Richard Von Sturmer, and Rodney Needham, trans. London: Eyre and Spottiswoode.

———. 1973 (Engl. trans.). *From Honey to Ashes*. John and Doreen Weightman, trans. New York: Harper and Row.

———. 1981 (Engl. trans.). *The Naked Man*. John Weightman and Doreen Weightman, trans. New York: Harper and Row.

———. 1983 [Engl. trans. 1969]. *The Raw and the Cooked*. John and Doreen Weightman, trans. Chicago: University of Chicago Press.

———. 1990 [Engl. trans. 1978]. *The Origin of Table Manners*, John and Doreen Weightman, trans. Chicago: University of Chicago Press.

Lispector, Clarice. 1988. *The Passion according to G.H.*, Ronald W. Sousa, trans. Minneapolis: University of Minnesota Press.

Livingstone, Frank B. 1962. "On the Non-existence of Human Races." *Current Anthropology* 3(3): 279–81.

———. 1963. "Comments on 'Geographic and Microgeographic Races' by Marshall T. Newman." *Current Anthropology* 4(2): 199–200.

Lock, Margaret. 2002 [2001]. "The Alienation of Body Tissue and the Biopolitics of Immortalized Cell Lines." In *Commodifying Bodies*, ed. Nancy Scheper-Hughes and Loïc Wacquant, 63–92. Thousand Oaks, CA: Sage Publications.

Lowitt, Mark H., and Neil Shear. 2001. "Pharmacogenomics and Dermatological Therapeutics." *Archives of Dermatology* 137(11): 1512–14.

Lowy, Ilana. 2000. "Trustworthy Knowledge and Desperate Patients: Clinical Tests for New Drugs from Cancer to AIDS." In *Living and Working with the New Medical Technologies: Intersections of Inquiry*, ed. Margaret Lock, Allan Young, and Alberto Cambrosio, 49–81. Cambridge: Cambridge University Press.

Marra, F., L. Lynd, M. Coombes, K. Richardson, M. Legal, J. M. Fitzgerald, and C. A. Marra. 2006. "Does Antibiotic Exposure during Infancy Lead to Development of Asthma? A Systematic Review and Metaanalysis." *Chest* 130(5): 1624.

Martin, Emily, and Richard A. Cone. n.d. Personal communication.

Masoudi, Frederick A., and Edward P. Havranek. 2001. "Letter to the Editor." *New England Journal of Medicine* 345(10): 767.

Massiah, Joycelin. 1986. "Work in the Lives of Caribbean Women." *Social and Economic Studies* 35(2): 177–240.

Maurer, Bill. 2000 [1997]. *Recharting the Caribbean: Land, Law, and Citizenship in the British Virgin Islands*. Ann Arbor: University of Michigan Press.

Mauss, Marcel. 1990 [1950]. *The Gift: The Form and Reason for Exchange in Archaic Societies*, W. D. Halls, trans. New York: W. W. Norton.

McConnell, W., and S. Holgate. 2000. "The Definition of Asthma: Its Relationship to Other Chronic Obstructive Lung Diseases." In *Asthma* (4th ed.), ed. T.J.H. Clark, S. Godfrey, T. H. Lee, and N. C. Thomson, 1–32. New York: Oxford University Press.

Miller, J. E. 2000. "The Effects of Race, Ethnicity, and Income on Early Childhood Asthma Prevalence and Health Care Use." *American Journal of Public Health* 90(3): 428–30.

Mintz, Sidney. 1985. *Sweetness and Power: The Place of Sugar in Modern History*. New York: Viking.

Mol, Annemarie. 1998. "Missing Links, Making Links: The Performance of Some Atheroscleroses." In *Differences in Medicine: Unraveling Practices, Techniques, and Bodies*, ed. Marc Berg and Annemarie Mol, 144–65. Durham: Duke University Press.

Montagu, Ashley. 1963a. "What Is Remarkable about Varieties of Man Is Likenesses, Not Differences." *Current Anthropology* 4(4): 361–64.

——. 1963b. "Regarding Montagu's Use of 'Ethnic Group.'" *American Anthropologist* 65(6): 1352–53.

——. 1997 [1942]. *Man's Most Dangerous Myth: The Fallacy of Race*. New York: Altamira Press.

Montoya, Michael J. 2007. "Bioethnic Conscription: Genes, Race, and Mexicana/o Ethnicity in Diabetes Research." *Cultural Anthropology* 22(1): 94–128.

Morahan, Grant, Dexing Huang, Mark Wu, Barbara J. Holt, Gregory P. White, Garth E. Kendall, Peter D. Sly, and Patrick G. Holt. 2002. "Association of IL12B Promoter Polymorphism with Severity of Atopic and Non-atopic Asthma in Children." *Lancet* 360: 455–59.

Munasinghe, Viranjini. 2006. "Theorizing World Culture through the New World: East Indians and Creolization." *American Ethnologist* 33(4): 549–62.

NAEPP (National Asthma Education and Prevention Program). n.d. "National Asthma Education and Prevention Program: Program Description." Unpublished pamphlet. Bethesda, MD: National Heart, Lung, and Blood Institute. www.nhlbi. nih.gov.

NCHS (National Center for Health Statistics). n.d. "Asthma Prevalence, Health Care Use and Mortality, 2000–2001." Unpublished pamphlet. Atlanta: Centers for Disease Control and Prevention. www.cdc.gov/nchs/products/pubs/pubd/hestats/asthma/asthma.htm.

Nelkin, Dorthy, and M. Susan Lindee. 1995. *The DNA Mystique: The Gene as a Cultural Icon.* New York: W. H. Freeman.

Nemesure, Barbara, Xiaodong Jiao, Qimei He, M. Cristina Leske, Suh-Yuh Wu, Anselm Hennis, Nancy Mendell, Joy Redman, Henri-Jean Garchon, Richa Agarwala, Alejandro A. Schaffer, Fielding Hejtmancik, and Barbados Family Study Group. 2003. "A Genome-Wide Scan for Primary Open Angle Glaucoma (POAG): The Barbados Family Study of Open Angle Glaucoma." *Human Genetics* 112 (5–6): 600–609.

Nickel, Renate G., Stephanie Ann Willadsen, Linda R. Freidhoff, Shau-Ku Huang, Luis Caraballo, Raana P. Naidu, Paul Levett, Malcolm Blumenthal, Susan Banks-Schlegel, Eugene Bleecker, Terri Beaty, Carole Ober, and Kathleen C. Barnes. 1999. "Determination of Duffy Genotypes in Three Populations of African Descent Using PCR and Sequence-Specific Oligonucleotides." *Human Immunology* 60: 738–42.

O'Connor, R. D., J. C. O'Donnell, L. A. Pinto, D. J. Wiener, and A. P. Legorreta. 2002. "Two Year Retrospective Economic Evaluation of Three Dual-Controller Therapies Used in the Treatment of Asthma." *Chest* 121(4): 1028–35.

Oldani, Michael. 2004. "Thick Prescriptions: Toward an Interpretation of Pharmaceutical Sales Practices." *Medical Anthropology Quarterly* 18(3): 325–56.

Olwig, Karen Fog. 1999. "The Burden of Heritage: Claiming a Place for a West Indian Culture." *American Ethnologist* 26(2): 370–88.

Omenn, Gilbert S., and Arno G. Motulsky. 2003. "Integration of Pharmacogenomics into Medical Practice." In *Pharmacogenomics: Social, Ethical and Clinical Dimensions,* ed. Mark A. Rothstein, 137–62. Hoboken, NJ: John Wiley.

Orta, Andrew. 2004. *Catechizing Culture: Missionaries, Aymara, and the "New Evangelization."* New York: Columbia University Press.

Palmié, Stephan. 2007. "Genomics, Divination, 'Racecraft.'" *American Ethnologist* 34(2): 205–22.

Pálsson, Gísli, and Paul Rabinow. 1999. "Iceland: The Case of a National Human Genome Project." *Anthropology Today* 15(2): 14–18.

———. 2005. "The Iceland Controversy: Reflections on the Transnational Market of Civic Virtue." In *Global Assemblages: Technology, Politics, and Ethics as Anthropological Problems,* ed. Aihwa Ong and Stephen J. Collier, 91–104. Malden, MA: Blackwell.

Peat, J. K., B. G. Toelle, G. B. Marks, and C. M. Mellis. 2001. "Continuing the Debate about Measuring Asthma in Population Studies." *Thorax* 56(5): 406–11.

Petryna, Adriana. 2002. *Life Exposed: Biological Citizens after Chernobyl.* Princeton: Princeton University Press.

———. 2005. "Ethical Variability: Drug Development and Globalizing Clinical Trials." *American Ethnologist* 32(2): 183–97.

Petryna, Adriana, Andrew Lakoff, and Arthur Kleinman, eds. 2006. *Global Pharmaceuticals: Ethics, Markets, Practices.* Durham: Duke University Press.

PhRMA. 2003. "PhRMA Comments/Recommendations on Guidance for Industry Collection of Race and Ethnicity Data in Clinical Trials." Unpublished pamphlet. www.phrma.org.

Pomerleau, J., P. M. McKeigue, and N. Chaturvedi. 1999. "Factors Associated with Obesity in South Asian, Afro-Caribbean and European Women." *International Journal of Obesity* 23: 25–33.

Pouillon, Jean. 1982 (Engl. trans.). "Remarks on the Verb 'To Believe.'" In *Between Belief and Transgression: Structuralist Essays in Religion, History, and Myth,* ed. Michel Izard and Pierre Smith, trans. John Leavitt, 1–9. Chicago: University of Chicago Press.

Prakash, Gyan. 1999. *Another Reason: Science and the Imagination of Modern India.* Princeton: Princeton University Press.

Price, M. J., and A. H. Briggs. 2002. "Development of an Economic Model to Assess the Cost Effectiveness of Asthma Management Strategies." *Pharmacoeconomics* 20(3): 183–94.

Puri, Shalini. 2003. "Beyond Resistance: Notes toward a New Caribbean Cultural Studies." *Small Axe* 14: 23–38.

———. 2004. "Commentary on 'Agricultural Hybridity and the 'Pathology' of Traditional Ways…' Developing Hybridities: A Response to Chris Shepherd." *Journal of Latin American Anthropology* 9(2): 273–77.

Rabinow, Paul. 1992. "Artificiality and Enlightenment: From Sociobiology to Biosociality." In *Incorporations, Zone 6,* ed. J. Crary and S. Kwinter, 234–52. Cambridge: MIT Press.

———. 1996. *Making PCR: A Story of Biotechnology.* Chicago: University of Chicago Press.

———. 1999. *French DNA: Trouble in Purgatory.* Chicago: University of Chicago Press.

Rahier, Jean Muteba. 2003. "Introduction: Mestizaje, Mulataje, Mestiçagem in Latin American Ideologies of National Identities." *Journal of Latin American Anthropology* 8(1): 40–51.

Rand, Cynthia S. 2002. "Adherence to Asthma Therapy in the Preschool Child." *Allergy* 57 (Suppl. 74): 48–57.

Rapp, Rayna. 1999. *Testing Women Testing the Fetus: The Social Impact of Amniocentesis in America.* New York: Routledge.

———. 2000. "Extra Chromosomes and Blue Tulips: Medico-Familial Interpretations." In *Living and Working with the New Medical Technologies: Intersections of Inquiry,* ed. Margaret Lock, Allan Young, and Alberto Cambrosio, 184–208. Cambridge: Cambridge University Press.

———. 2003. "Cell Life and Death, Child Life and Death: Genomic Horizons, Genetic Diseases, Family Stories." In *Remaking Life and Death: Toward an Anthropology of the Biosciences,* ed. Sarah Franklin and Margaret Lock, 129–64. Santa Fe: School of American Research Press.

Reardon, Jenny. 2005. *Race to the Finish: Identity and Governance in an Age of Genomics.* Princeton: Princeton University Press.

Reddel, Helen, Sandra Ware, Guy Marks, Cheryl Salome, Christine Jenkins, and Ann Woolcock. 1999. "Differences between Asthma Exacerbations and Poor Asthma Control." *Lancet* 353: 364–69.

Reilly, Philip R. 2001. "Legal Issues in Genomic Medicine." *Nature Medicine* 7(3): 268–71.

Robotham, Don. 1996. "Transnationalism in the Caribbean: Formal and Informal." *American Ethnologist* 25(2): 307–21.

Romualdi, Chiara, David Balding, Ivane S. Nasidze, Gregory Risch, Myles Robichaux, Stephen T. Sherry, Mark Stoneking, Mark A. Batzer, and Guido Barbujani. 2002. "Patterns of Human Diversity, within and among Continents, Inferred from Biallelic DNA Polymorphisms." *Genome Research* 12: 602–12.

Rona, Roberto J. 2000. "Asthma and Poverty." *Thorax* 55: 239–44.

Rose, Nikolas, and Carlos Novas. 2005. "Biological Citizenship." In *Global Assemblages: Technology, Politics, and Ethics as Anthropological Problems*, ed. Aihwa Ong and Stephen J. Collier, 439–63. Malden, MA: Blackwell.

Rosenberg, Noah A., Jonathan K. Pritchard, James L. Weber, Howard M. Cann, Kenneth K. Kidd, Lev A. Zhivotovsky, and Marcus W. Feldman. 2002. "Genetic Structure of Human Populations." *Science* 298: 2381–85.

Rothstein, Mark A., ed. 2003. *Pharmacogenomics: Social, Ethical and Clinical Dimensions*. Hoboken, NJ: John Wiley.

Rothstein, Mark A., and Phyllis Griffin Epps. 2001. "Ethical and Legal Implications of Pharmacogenomics." *Nature Reviews Genetics* 2: 228–31.

Rowley, Michelle. 2002. "Reconceptualizing Voice: The Role of Matrifocality in Shaping Theories and Caribbean Voices." In *Gendered Realities: Essays in Caribbean Feminist Thought*, ed. Patricia Mohammed, 22–33. Kingston, Jamaica: University of the West Indies Press.

Rusnak, James M., Robert M. Kisabeth, David P. Herbert, and Dennis M. McNeil. 2001. "Pharmacogenomics: A Clinician's Primer on Emerging Technologies for Improved Patient Care." *Mayo Clinic Proceedings* 76: 299–309.

Safa, Helen. 2005. "The Matrifocal Family and Patriarchal Ideology in Cuba and the Caribbean." *Journal of Latin American Anthropology* 10(2): 314–38.

Salter, Henry Hyde. 1860. *On Asthma: Its Pathology and Treatment*. London: John Churchil.

Sapp, Jan. 1983. "The Struggle for Authority in the Field of Heredity, 1900–1932: New Perspectives on the Rise of Genetics." *Journal of the History of Biology* 16(3): 311–42.

Scheper-Hughes, Nancy. 1992. "*Nervoso*: Medicine, Sickness, and Human Needs." In *Death without Weeping: The Violence of Everyday Life in Brazil*, 167–215. Berkeley: University of California Press.

Schwartz, Michael. 1952. *Heredity in Bronchial Asthma: A Clinical and Genetic Study of 191 Asthma Probands and 50 Probands with Baker's Asthma*. Acta Allergologica 5 (Suppl. II). Copenhagen: Ejnar Munskgaard.

Segal, Daniel A. 1993. "'Race' and 'Colour' in Pre-independence Trinidad and Tobago." In *Trinidad Ethnicity*, ed. Kevin Yelvington, 81–115. Knoxville: University of Tennessee Press.

Segal, Daniel A. 2006. "Circulation, Transpositions, and the Travails of Creole." *American Ethnologist* 33(4): 579–81.

Sell, Susan. 2003. *Private Power, Public Law: The Globalization of Intellectual Property Rights.* Cambridge: Cambridge University Press.

Senior, Olive. 1991. *Working Miracles: Women's Lives in the English-Speaking Caribbean.* Bloomington: Indiana University Press.

Shanawani, H., L. Dame, D. A. Schwartz, and R. Cook-Deegan. 2006. "Non-reporting and Inconsistent Reporting of Race and Ethnicity in Articles That Claim Associations among Genotype, Outcome, and Race or Ethnicity." *Journal of Medical Ethics* 32(12): 724–28.

Shapiro, Steven D., and Caroline A. Owen. 2002. "ADAM-33 Surfaces as an Asthma Gene." *New England Journal of Medicine* 347(12): 936–38.

Shields, Alexandra E., Michael Fortun, Evelynn M. Hammonds, Patricia A. King, Caryn Lerman, Rayna Rapp, and Patrick F. Sullivan. 2005. "The Use of Race Variables in Genetic Studies of Complex Traits and the Goal of Reducing Health Disparities: A Transdisciplinary Perspective." *American Psychologist* 60(1): 77–103.

Smedley, Brian D., Adrienne Y. Stith, and Alan R. Nelson, eds. 2003. *Unequal Treatment: Confronting Racial and Ethnic Disparities in Healthcare.* Washington, DC: Institute of Medicine of the National Academies.

Spencer, Kevin, Charas Y. T. Ong, Adolfo W. J. Liao, and Kypros H. Nicolaides. 2000. "The Influence of Ethnic Origin on First Trimester Biochemical Markers of Chromosomal Abnormalities." *Prenatal Diagnosis* 20: 491–94.

Steiner, George. 1998 [1975]. *After Babel: Aspects of Language and Translation* (3rd ed.). New York: Oxford University Press.

Stepan, Nancy. 1982. *The Idea of Race in Science.* Hamden, CT: Archon Books.

Stephens, J. Claiborne, Julie A. Schneider, Debra A. Tanguay, Julie Choi, Tara Acharya, Scott E. Stanley, Ruhong Jiang, Chad J. Messer, Anne Chew, Jin-Hua Han, Jicheng Duan, Janet L. Carr, Min Seob Lee, Beena Koshy, A. Madan Kumar, Ge Zhang, William R. Newell, Andreas Windemuth, Chuanbo Xu, Theodore S. Kalbfleish, Sandra L. Shaner, Kevin Arnold, Vincent Schulz, Connie M. Drysdale, Krishnan Nandabalan, Richard S. Judson, Gualberto Ruano, and Gerald F. Vovis. 2001. "Haplotype Variation and Linkage Disequilibrium in 313 Human Genes." *Science* 293: 489–93.

Stocking, George W., Jr. 1982 [1968]. *Race, Culture, and Evolution: Essays in the History of Anthropology.* Chicago: University of Chicago Press.

Stoler, Ann Laura. 1995. *Race and the Education of Desire: Foucault's History of Sexuality and the Colonial Order of Things.* Durham: Duke University Press.

Strathern, Marilyn. 1980. "No Nature, No Culture: The Hagen Case." In *Nature, Culture and Gender,* ed. Carol P. McCormack and Marilyn Strathern, 174–222. New York: Cambridge University Press.

Sutton, Constance, and Susan Makiesky-Barrow. 1977. "Social Inequality and Sexual Status in Barbados." In *Sexual Stratification: A Cross-Cultural View,* ed. Alice Schlegel, 293–325. New York: Columbia University Press.

Tattersfield, A. E., A. J. Knox, J. R. Britton, and I. P. Hall. 2002. "Asthma." *Lancet* 360(9342): 1313–22.

Taussig, Karen-Sue, Rayna Rapp, and Deborah Heath. 2003. "Flexible Eugenics: Technologies of the Self in the Age of Genetics." In *Genetic Nature/Culture: Anthropology beyond the Two-Culture Divide*, ed. Alan H. Goodman, Deborah Heath, and M. Susan Lindee, 58–76. Berkeley: University of California Press.

Temple, Robert. 2002. "Policy Developments in Regulatory Approval." *Statistics in Medicine* 21: 2939–48.

Thomas, Deborah. 2004. *Modern Blackness: Nationalism, Globalization, and the Politics of Culture in Jamaica*. Durham: Duke University Press.

Thorowgood, John C. 1870. *Notes on Asthma: Its Nature, Forms, and Treatment*. London: John Churchill.

Trostle, James. 1996. "Introduction: Inappropriate Distribution of Medicines by Professionals in Developing Countries." *Social Science and Medicine* 42(8): 1117–20.

Ungar, Wendy J., Kenneth R. Chapman, and Maria T. Santos. 2002. "Assessment of a Medication-Based Asthma Index for Population Research." *American Journal of Respiratory and Critical Care Medicine* 165(2): 190–94.

Wailoo, Keith. 1997. *Drawing Blood: Technology and Disease Identity in Twentieth-Century America*. Baltimore: Johns Hopkins University Press.

Wailoo, Keith, and Stephen Pemberton. 2006. *The Troubled Dream of Genetic Medicine: Ethnicity and Innovation in Tay-Sachs, Cystic Fibrosis, and Sickle Cell Disease*. Baltimore: Johns Hopkins University Press.

Warren, Kay B. 2001. "Introduction: Rethinking Bi-polar Constructions of Ethnicity." *Journal of Latin American Anthropology* 6(2): 90–105.

Weinstein, Andrew G., Bruce Bender, Andrea Apter, Henry Milgrom, Lisa Kobrynski, and Paul Williams. n.d. "Achieving Adherence to Asthma Therapy." Unpublished AAAAI Quality of Care for Asthma Committee Paper. Milwaukee, WI: American Academy of Allergy, Asthma and Immunology (AAAAI).

Wellcome Trust Case Control Consortium. 2007. "Genome-Wide Association Study of 14,000 Cases of Seven Common Diseases and 3,000 Shared Controls." *Nature* 447: 661–78.

Westermann, Cornelius J. J., Ahlsen F. Rosina, Vanessa de Vries, and Pamela A. de Coteau. 2003. "The Prevalence and Manifestations of Hereditary Hemorrhagic Telangiectasia in the Afro-Caribbean Population of the Netherlands Antilles: A Family Screening." *American Journal of Medical Genetics* 116A: 324–28.

Whyte, Susan Reynolds, Sjaak van der Geest, and Anita Hardon. 2002. *Social Lives of Medicines*. Cambridge: Cambridge University Press.

Wilson, James F., Michael E. Weale, Alice C. Smith, Fiona Gratrix, Benjamin Fletcher, Mark G. Thomas, Neil Bradman, and David B. Goldstein. 2001. "Population Genetic Structure of Variable Drug Response." *Nature Genetics* 29(3): 265–69.

Worboys, Michael. 1999. "Tuberculosis and Race in Britain and Its Empire, 1900–1950." In *Race, Science, and Medicine, 1700–1960*, ed. Waltraud Ernst and Bernard Harris, 144–66. New York: Routledge.

Xu, Jianfeng, Deborah A. Meyers, Carole Ober, Malcolm N. Blumenthal, Beverly Mellen, Kathleen C. Barnes, Richard A. King, Lucille A. Lester, Timothy D. Howard, Julian Solway, Carl D. Langefeld, Terri H. Beaty, Stephen S. Rich, Eugene R.

Bleecker, Nancy J. Cox, and the Collaborative Study on the Genetics of Asthma. 2001. "Genomewide Screen and Identification of Gene-Gene Interactions for Asthma-Susceptibility Loci in Three U.S. Populations: Collaborative Study on the Genetics of Asthma." *American Journal of Human Genetics* 68: 1437–46.

Yelvington, Kevin, ed. 1993. *Trinidad Ethnicity.* Knoxville: University of Tennessee Press.

Index

acute lung injury genetics, 33, 98–101, 103–4, 113, 198

ADAM33, 67, 171–72, 197

adherence and nonadherence: anthropology of, 87–88; and medical care, 9, 11, 55, 70, 75, 81, 87–92, 94–95, 185; as research focus, 65–66; and side effects, 55, 89–92. *See also* irrational patient

adrenaline, 3, 61, 64, 100–101

Adult Respiratory Health Questionnaire, 159–64, 166–69

Africa, 17, 24–25, 102, 109–10, 113–14, 167–68, 200n2, 200n3

African Americans: and asthma, 5, 22, 29–32; and Bajans, 7, 12, 30, 33, 114–16, 164, 168, 171–73; and genetic research, 5, 7, 16–18, 22–23, 25, 29–32, 113–16, 166–68, 171–73, 194n10; and heart disease, 28–29

African ancestry, heritage, origin, 17–18, 25, 30–31, 112–16, 164–69, 171–72, 200n3, 200–201n4

Afro-Caribbean as race/ethnicity, 12, 33, 116, 123, 164, 166–69, 172

Afro-Trinidadian as race/ethnicity, 199–200n2, 200–201n4, 202n12

air filters, 110, 173, 179

allergen test, 65, 118, 176–82, 187, 201–2n11

allergy shots, 61, 66

ambivalence, 14, 36, 42–44, 54–55, 81, 97, 108, 147–48, 187–89

ambulances, 76, 148–49, 154

American Anthropological Association, 33

Americanization. *See* U.S., views of

Amish, 171, 173

anomalies, 13–14, 132–33, 179, 202n1

anonymity, 195n1

antibiotics, 44–45, 75–76, 94–95, 125, 128

antihistamines, 102, 125

Arnold, David, 103

asbestos, 199n9

Asian as race/ethnicity, 25–26, 112–13, 164–65

asthma: cause of, 3, 11, 65–66, 82–87, 108–11, 133–39, 162–64, 183–84; diagnosis of, 70–76, 101, 106–7, 120–24; genetics of, 4–6, 29–30, 61–64, 67–68; history of, 56–64; patient perspectives on, 119–24, 145–46, 160–61, 181–82; prevalence of, 2, 9, 36, 69–75, 100, 102, 107, 119–20; public health intervention on, 35–36, 76–81, 94–97, 105–6; racial disparities in, 22, 29–32, 102, 114–15; variability of, 3, 64–68, 159–62. *See also* genetics: and asthma

asthma pharmaceuticals: combination inhalers, 37, 55, 66–67, 70, 90, 92–96; inhaled steroids, 37–38, 66, 70, 82, 87–92, 95–97, 127; long-acting $\beta2$ agonists, 66–67,

asthma pharmaceuticals *(continued)*
92–94; oral steroids, 64, 66, 70, 87, 90–91,
126–27, 132–33; overprescription of, 75–76,
95–96, 124–25, 129, 132–33; short-acting
β2 agonists, 48, 65–66, 70, 72, 131, 196–97n5;
side effects, 126–28; use for diagnosis, 3,
71–73, 65, 67, 196–97n5, 197n6
asthma severity, 3, 29–31, 65–67, 159–60
asthma traditional treatments, 120, 127,
129–31
AstraZeneca, 41, 67, 80, 92–94, 103, 195
atopy, 6, 61–65, 105, 107, 115, 159, 172–173
Avruch, Kevin, 200n2

Baltimore, 102, 168, 172
Barbadian v. Bajan, 192n5
Barbados: ethnic identities in, 7, 112–13,
154–69; gender in, 146, 149; genetic
research in, 1–2, 6–10, 33–35, 97–99,
185, 201n8; health care system, 7, 33–36;
immigration and emigration, 112, 154,
165. *See also* Caribbean: Barbados's
position in
Barbados Asthma Genetics Study: design,
1–2, 6, 30–32, 34, 98–103, 118, 157–70,
174–75, 179–80; recruitment, 34, 139–41,
145; results, 6, 103–4, 109, 114, 160,
168, 171–73
Barrow, Christine, 146
Bateson, Gregory, 45, 188, 202n2
Beck, Ulrich, 92
Becotide, 95–96
Berotec, 32, 72, 176
β2 adrenergic receptor gene, 30, 67, 197n6
Bhabha, Homi, 193n4, 202n12
BiDil, 15, 28–29
Biehl, João, 8, 39, 119
biomedicalization, 9, 11, 14, 181–82
biotechnology industry, 4–7, 15, 17, 67
blood, 19–20, 56–58, 64, 157–58, 174–75
blood pressure, 35, 54, 102, 106, 113–14
Blumenbach, Johann Friedrich, 194
Boas, Franz, 20–21
Boon, James, 14, 32, 117, 143, 172, 188,
197n2, 207n12
Brandt, Allan, 197–98n6
Braun, Lundy, 201n7
Brazil, 8, 39, 44, 88, 114, 200n2
Bridgetown, 35–36
Briggs, Charles, 197n6
bronchitis, 70, 73
Buffon, Georges-Louis Leclerc de, 21
Bulmer, Ralph, 23, 192–93n11
bush teas. *See* asthma traditional treatments

Canada, 72, 128, 149
cancer genetics, 15, 33, 35, 53–54, 106,
114–16, 186
Caribbean: Barbados's position in, 35, 39,
43, 48–50, 53, 154, 199n8; gender in,
146–49; internationalism in, 54, 143, 196;
pharmaceutical industry in, 43, 48, 90–91;
race in, 112, 164–67, 198–200
Carnival, 166, 201n6
Caucasian as race/ethnicity, 5, 15–18, 26, 33,
112–14, 164–69, 171–72, 194n6, 194n8,
198n3, 199–200n2, 200n4
Centers for Disease Control and Prevention,
29, 159
centrifuge, 201n8
Chicago, 102, 168
chicken, 85, 109, 137, 162
Childhood Asthma Management Program, 67
Chinese as race/ethnicity, 112, 164–65
chlordane, 138–39
chloroform, 59–60
Chronic Disease Research Center, 34, 55
cigarettes, 59, 65, 109, 134, 179, 198n7, 162–63
cleaning products, 65, 85
clinical trials, 16, 24–26, 102, 191n2, 192n6
cockroaches, 31, 65, 82, 159, 162, 176–77
Collaborative Study on Genetics of Asthma,
5, 30–32, 166–68, 172, 180
colonialism, 47–48, 164, 193n4, 193–94n5,
199n2, 199n8
Columbia, 178
compliance. *See* adherence
compulsory licensing, 45–46
Cone, Richard, 199n7
conferences in Barbados, 54, 80, 92–94, 103–4,
109–15
Consortium to Evaluate Lung Edema
Genetics, 100
consuming modernity, 86
contract research organizations, 24, 26
contradiction, 2, 12–14, 32, 52, 117, 165–66,
169, 180–84, 187–89
Cooke, Robert A., 62–64
Coon, Carleton, 21
Count, Earl, 21
Crop–Over, 165–66
Current Anthropology, 20–21
Cuvier, Georges, 194n12
CYP 450 complex, 25–26, 30

Das, Ranendra, 87–88, 195–96n3
Das, Veena, 87–88, 195–96n3
databases, 8, 10, 24, 30, 100, 113, 171–73, 180,
186, 192n4, 197n7

DeCODE, 5, 67, 171–72, 197n6, 197n7
dengue fever, 33, 85–86, 98–101, 105–6
diabetes, 22, 26, 35, 105–6, 114, 116
DNA, 100, 113, 158, 174
Dobzhansky, Theodosius, 21–22
Douglas, Mary, 13, 184
drug metabolism. See CYP 450 complex
Drug Service Committees, 37–53, 55
Du Bois, W.E.B., 194n7
duffy genotype, 168
dust, Bajan meaning of, 12, 84, 109, 112, 128,
  133–35, 154, 163, 183–84, 201n7
Duster, Troy, 194n10, 195n13
dust from Africa. See Sahara dust

emergency room. See Queen Elizabeth
  Hospital: Accident and Emergency
  Department
endotoxins, 109, 114–15, 162
England, 7, 33, 43, 47–48, 129–30
environment as category: in Barbados, 52,
  82–86, 105–6; in genetic research, 22, 29–32,
  102, 108–11, 115–16, 162–64, 172–73,
  179–80. See also pollution
environmental health officials, 83–86
eosinophils, 65, 184
epidemiologists, 3, 6, 29, 67, 159, 201n8
Ernst, Waltraud, 18, 193n4
ethnic correction, 166
evolutionary history, 17, 114, 195n12, 196n4

family as category: in Barbados, 146, 158, 167,
  199n1; in genetic research, 19, 34, 62–64,
  122, 129–41, 169–70, 174; in medicine, 52,
  71, 74–75, 80–81, 132–33
Farmer, Paul, 88
Floyer, Sir John, 56–57, 61–62, 196n2
food and asthma, 47, 57–58, 60, 65, 82, 84–86,
  111, 134–39
Food and Drug Administration, 4, 6, 15–16,
  24–26, 28–29, 37
Formulary Committee. See Drug Service
  Committees
Foster, Morris, 15
Foucault, Michel, 27–28, 57, 94, 193n3, 193n4,
  195n12, 196n2
Freeman, Carla, 34, 146, 192n5, 199n2
Fullwiley, Duana, 17
futurism, 103–4, 117, 185–88

Gabbert, Wolfgang, 200n2
garlic water. See asthma traditional treatments
Gaudillière, Jean-Paul, 62
Genaissance, 17–18, 67

generic pharmaceuticals, 37, 40–42, 45–47
genetic counselors, 105, 201
geneticization, 19, 97, 189
genetic research: ambivalence toward, 54–55,
  97, 105–8, 111, 139–44; as arcane, 12, 74–75,
  115–16, 142–44, 174–75; on common
  diseases, 4, 98; facilitation of, 98–103,
  157–58; and nationhood, 8, 34–35, 53–54;
  speed and scale of, 99–100, 103–4, 108
Genome Therapeutics, 67, 171
Genomic Research in African American
  Pedigrees Project, 21
genotyping technologies, 99, 104, 107,
  109–10, 116–17
gift logic, 41–42, 53, 76–79, 103, 117, 132
Gilroy, Paul, 200n3, 202n12
glaucoma, 26, 33, 53–54, 90, 102, 116
GlaxoSmithKline, 51–52, 59, 67, 73, 77, 90, 96
Global Initiative for Asthma, 101
global markets, 8, 23–24, 39, 42–55, 83–87,
  117, 186–87
Good, Byron, 198n1
Good, Mary Jo Delvecchio, 198n1
Guyanese as race/ethnicity, 112, 164–65, 167

Haplotype Map, 23–24
Harlem, 31–32
Harrison, Faye, 21, 194n7
heart medication, 15–16, 25, 28–29, 55
heredity, 19, 60–64, 74–75, 123–24, 179, 196n4
Hispanic as race/ethnicity, 22, 27, 29–31, 113,
  166–67
HIV/AIDS, 39, 44, 54, 79, 88, 155, 198n3
Hoetnik, H., 200n3
hospital. See Queen Elizabeth Hospital
Howard University, 22
Howitt, Malcolm, 69
human genome, 16, 171, 180
Human Genome Diversity Project, 195n14
Human Genome Project, 15, 103
hybridity, 165, 180, 200–201n4, 202n12
hygiene hypothesis, 3, 115–16
Hymes, Dell, 202n7
hyperdiagnostics, 26–27, 184–85

Iceland, 5, 8, 34, 197. See also DeCODE
immunoglobin E levels, 65, 67, 159–60, 171
immunologists, 61, 201n10
Indian as race/ethnicity, 25, 112, 164–66,
  200–201n4
individualization, 16, 52, 93, 116, 153–54,
  195n13, 197–98n6
Indo-Trinidadian as race/ethnicity, 199n2,
  200n4, 202n12

International Monetary Fund, 44, 82, 196n4
International Study on Asthma and Allergies
    in Childhood, 69, 107
irrational patient, 87–92, 96

Jackson, Mark, 194n5
Jamaica, 35, 54
James, Deborah, 200n2
Johns Hopkins University, 1–2, 6, 30, 33, 98
Journal of the American Medical Association, 16

Kahn, Jonathan, 15, 28
Keirns, Carla, 57–61, 64, 196n1
Kevles, Daniel, 19–20
Khan, Aisha, 165, 198n3, 199n2, 200n4, 202n12

Lancet, 3, 16
Latour, Bruno, 104
Lee, Sandra, 16
Lesser, Jeffrey, 200n2
leukotriene receptor antagonists, 30,
    66–67, 107
Lévi-Strauss, Claude, 13, 94, 103, 139, 180,
    188, 198–99n6, 199n10, 201–2n11, 202n2,
    203n4
Linnaeus, Carolus von, 21, 27
Lispector, Clarice, 203n5
literacy rate, 34–35
Livingstone, Frank, 20–22, 194n9
lizard soup. *See* asthma traditional treatments
Lock, Margaret, 10
Löwy, Ilana, 62

marketization, 50–51, 76–77
Martin, Emily, 199n7
Maurer, Bill, 201n5
Mauss, Marcel, 79, 188
Medco Research, 28
Merck, 46
metabolic syndrome, 114
methacholine, 65, 67, 159–60, 196–97n5, 199n1
Mintz, Sidney, 199n8
modernization, 82–87, 97, 115, 133–39,
    162–64, 183–84
Mol, Annemarie, 202n8
Montagu, Ashley, 21, 194n8
motherhood: and asthma, 61, 63; and genetic
    research, 11–12, 139–41, 145, 154–56,
    175–76; as medical responsibility, 11, 88–89,
    145–53, 187–88
myths, 13, 21, 180, 188, 192n7

N-acetyltransferase 2 gene, 26–27
National Asthma Education and Prevention
    Program, 66

National Drug Formulary, 35–53, 70, 81, 92,
    95–96
National Heart, Lung, and Blood Institute,
    2, 4, 6, 66
National Human Genome Research Institute,
    23–24
National Institutes of Health, 4, 15–16, 23–24,
    54, 90–91, 192n3
nationalism and internationalism, 8, 39, 51–55,
    185, 196n6
National Library of Medicine, 196n1
Nature, 16, 108
nature/culture distinction, 13, 50, 139
nebulizers, 88, 121, 140
New England Journal of Medicine, 16
New York Times, 67
NitroMed, 28
nonadherence. *See* adherence
Novas, Carlos, 8

obesity, 33, 114
obstructive sleep apnea, 33, 98–103, 113–14
Office of Management and Budget, 23–25
Oldani, Michael, 40
Olwig, Karen, 200n3
Organization of Eastern Caribbean States,
    48–49, 54
Orta, Andrew, 198n5

Pan American Health Organization, 86
patents, 37, 39–40, 45–47, 67, 92, 95–96.
    See also pharmaceutical industry
peak airflow meters, 71–73
Peat, J. K., 3
pesticides. *See* pollution
Petryna, Adriana, 10
pharmaceutical citizen, 87–89, 94, 96
pharmaceutical industry: and asthma
    diagnosis, 13, 65–67, 69–73, 76–78; in
    Barbados, 8–9, 35–47, 92–94; marketing
    and education, 76–82; as moral/immoral,
    41–42, 45–46, 78, 198n7
pharmaceuticalization, 8–9, 14, 39, 53, 81–82,
    86–87, 96–97, 187
pharmacies, 35, 131–32
pharmacoeconomics, 65, 94
pharmacogenomics, 4–6, 17, 65, 191n1, 191n2,
    191–92n3, 197n6
PhRMA, 25–26
pollution, 3, 9, 65, 82–87, 110, 133–39, 179,
    183–84
polyclinics, 35–36, 69–72, 77–79, 151–52
Poole, Deborah, 195–96n3
population genetics, 16–18, 20, 201n8
Portuguese as race/ethnicity, 167, 199n2

potential asthmatic, 73–76, 97, 122–23, 186
Pouillon, Jean, 203n3
Prakash, Gyan, 193n4
predisposition, 1, 4–5, 15, 26, 31, 33, 62–64, 172, 185
prestige, 92, 99
preventer inhalers. *See* asthma pharmaceuticals: long-acting β2 agonists, combination inhalers, and inhaled steroids
psychoanalysis, 61
Puerto Rico, 121, 162
Pulmicort, 37, 80, 91, 96
pulmonology, 61, 64–65
Puri, Shalini, 201n6

Queen Elizabeth Hospital, 35–36, 44–45, 81, 88–89; Accident and Emergency Department, 70, 87–88, 100–102, 132, 139–40, 145, 150–53; Asthma Bay, 36, 88–89, 100–102, 152

race in science and medicine: as contested, 5–6, 15–16; as contradictory, 1–2, 6, 12–13, 17–18, 26–28, 166–69, 182, 184, 187; FDA on, 24–26; history of, 18–20; as moral issue, 20–22, 31–32, 113–15, 171–72, 185; NIH on, 23–24; pharmaceutical industry on, 25–29; as proxy, 29, 172–73, 180
Rapp, Rayna, 10, 119
rationality, 39, 61, 72, 88–89
Reardon, Jenny, 16, 20, 30, 32, 195n14
reflexivity, 7, 14, 27–28, 39, 50, 97, 189
reliever inhalers: *See* asthma pharmaceuticals: short-acting β2 agonists
risk, 88, 92, 197–98n6
roadwork. *See* pollution
Robotham, Don, 196n4, 196n6, 200n3
Rose, Nikolas, 8
Rowley, Michelle, 148, 153
rural v. urban health care, 71, 81

Sahara dust, 99, 110, 134
Salter, Henry Hyde, 57–63
Sapp, Jan, 196n4
Scheper-Hughes, Nancy, 88
Schering-Plough, 67, 171–72
schismogenesis, 45–47, 188
Science, 17
science as language, 27–28, 172, 181
Segal, Daniel, 165, 200–201n4
Senior, Olive, 146
sepsis, 100–101
September 11th attacks, 47
Seretide, 67, 90, 92

Shanawani, H. L., 23
Sharp, Richard, 15
Shields, Alexandra, 16
Shriver, Mark, 17
sickle cell anemia, 16, 19, 20, 22, 63, 193n2
single nucleotide polymorphisms, 103, 113
skin prick test. *See* allergen test
spirometry, 7, 159–61, 196–97n5, 201n7
Steiner, George, 181, 202n1
Stepan, Nancy, 18, 195n12
Stoler, Ann, 193n4
Strathern, Marilyn, 199n10
structuralism, 180, 188
sugar industry, 36, 47–48, 82, 136–37, 183, 199n8, 109
SUNY Stony Brook, 33, 116
Symbicort, 37, 55, 92, 95, 195n2

Taussig, Karen Sue, 10
Tenders Committee. *See* Drug Service Committees
Thomas, Deborah, 198n3
Thorax, 3
tourism, 46–47, 82, 200n3
Trade-Related Aspects of Intellectual Property Rights, 39, 44–45
transparency, 52–53
Trinidad, 164–65, 198n3, 200–201n4
tuberculosis, 22, 26, 60, 88, 193n5
Tuskegee Study, 20

United States, perspectives on, 46–48, 51–52, 109, 112, 130–31, 136, 139, 142–44
United States Census Bureau, 23
University of California at San Francisco, 30
University of Southampton, 67
University of the West Indies, 69, 102

Vander Veer, Albert, 62–64
vehicle exhaust. *See* pollution
Venter, Craig, 16
Ventolin, 73, 87, 95, 124, 130, 142, 152, 176
vernaculars, 2, 14, 169, 182, 202n12

Wailoo, Keith, 19–20, 59, 63, 193n2
Warren, Kay, 199–200n2
Washington, D.C., 4–6
Weber, Max, 89
wheeze, 56, 65, 70–73, 95, 97, 119–22, 151, 159–60
white as race/ethnicity. *See* Caucasian as race/ethnicity
Worboys, Michael, 193–94n5, 194n6
World Bank, 44
World Trade Organization, 44, 82